Student Nurse Thomas J. Bean
Cleybury Hospital.

Care of the Mentally Ill

Student Nurse Thomas J. Bean
Cleybury Hospital.

Care of the Mentally Ill

Peggy Martin

SECOND EDITION

MACMILLAN

First published 1983
Reprinted (with corrections) 1984 (twice)
Second edition 1987

Published by
MACMILLAN EDUCATION LTD
Houndmills, Basingstoke, Hampshire RG21 2XS
and London
Companies and representatives throughout the world.

ISBN 0 333 44080 3

Printed in Great Britain by
Scotprint Ltd, Musselburgh, Scotland

For my mother

Contents

Foreword to the series

This series of textbooks offers a fresh approach to the study of nursing. The aim is to give those beginning a career in nursing, and those already qualified, opportunities for reflection in order to broaden their approach to nursing education and to identify their own nursing values. The text includes material currently required by those preparing for qualification as a nurse and offers a basis for developing knowledge by individual studies. It should also assist qualified nurses returning to nursing and those wishing to gain further insight into the nursing curriculum.

The authors of each book in the series are from widely differing nursing backgrounds, and, as experienced teachers of nursing or midwifery, they are well aware of the difficulties faced by nursing students searching for meaning from a mass of factual information. The nurse has to practise in the real world, and in reality nursing students need to learn to practise with confidence and understanding. The authors have therefore collaborated to illustrate this new perspective by making full use of individual nursing care plans to present the knowledge required by the nursing student in the most appropriate and relevant way. These textbooks can therefore be used in a wide variety of nursing programmes.

The practice of nursing—as a profession and as a career—and the education of the nurse to fulfil her role are both affected by national and international trends. The Nurses, Midwives and Health Visitors Act 1979 in the United Kingdom, the Treaty of Rome and the European Community Nursing Directives 1977, as well as the deliberations and publications of the International Council of Nurses and the World Health Organization, all make an impact upon the preparation and the practice of the nurse throughout the world.

Nursing values may not have changed over the past hundred years, but society and both the patterns of life and care have changed, and are constantly changing. It is particularly important, therefore, to restate the essentials of nursing in the light of current practice and future trends.

Throughout this series the focus is on nursing and on the individual—the person requiring care and the person giving care—and emphasises the need for continuity between home and hospital care. *Neighbourhood Nursing—A Focus for Care*—the Report of the Community Nursing Review under the chairmanship of Julia Cumberlege (HMSO, 1986) has drawn attention to this need. The developing role of the nurse in primary care and in health education is reflected throughout this series. The authors place their emphasis on the whole person, and nursing care studies and care plans are used to promote understanding of the clinical, social, psychological and spiritual aspects of care for the individual.

Each book introduces the various aspects of the curriculum for general nursing: the special needs of (1) those requiring acute care; (2) the elderly; (3) children; (4) the mentally ill; and (5) the mentally handicapped. The latter is a new text in *The Essentials of Nursing Series*, edited by a well-known and respected nurse for the mentally handicapped and with contributors experienced in differing aspects of caring for people with mental handicap. The text on maternity and neonatal care, written by a midwifery teacher, provides the material for nursing students and would be helpful to those undertaking preparation for further health-visiting education.

The authors wish to acknowledge their gratitude for the assistance they have received from members of the Editorial Board, and from all those who have contributed to their work—patients and their relatives, students, qualified nurses and colleagues too numerous to mention by name. To all those nurse teachers who have read some of the texts, offering constructive criticism and comment from their special knowledge, we offer our grateful thanks. Lastly, we thank Elizabeth Horne, for her contribution to the physiology material in the text, and Mary Waltham for her help with this second edition.

1987   Sheila Collins

Preface

This book is written primarily for the general nursing student who is undertaking psychiatric nursing experience. The aim of the book is to introduce the learner to his or her role in caring for patients using individual patients problems and different approaches to nursing intervention within the psychiatric care setting. The second edition of *Care of the Mentally Ill* introduces the nursing student to the use of nursing models; two models are discussed in the Introduction and the practical application of these models is illustrated in Chapter 1 entitled Nursing the Patient who is Anxious. Readers may decide for themselves which model they would prefer to use. The choice of a model for nursing practice will depend on the appropriateness for the individual patient, the care setting, as well as the nurse's knowledge, familiarity and confidence in using a particular model.

Each chapter begins with an introduction to an emotional or behavioural problem; this is followed by a patient profile and a problem-orientated approach to care.

This textbook provides a basic foundation on which the nursing student can build and extend his or her knowledge. This series of books has been designed in such a way that the learner can add notes from observations, lectures and further study. A list of further reading is included at the end of each chapter.

1987   P.M.

Acknowledgements

I should like to express my thanks to the following people: Mary Waltham, Publisher of nursing books at Macmillan Education, for seeing this second edition through; Sheila Collins, Edith Parker, David Sharpe, Reg Everest and all the members of the Editorial Board for their encouragement; Geoff Bourne for reading the new material and making helpful and constructive comments; Peter Pocock for allowing me to use the diagram on page 6. Finally, thanks are due to Doris Crouch for typing the manuscript and to my husband Graham for his support.

A note on the series style

Throughout this book, in keeping with the other titles in this series, the term *nursing student* has been used to mean *both* student or pupil nurses *and* trained nurses who are undertaking post-basic training or who are keeping up to date with the recent literature. For clarity and consistency throughout the series the nurse is described as *she;* this is done without prejudice to men who are nurses or nursing students. Similarly, the patient is sometimes referred to as *he,* when the gender is not specifically mentioned.

Care plans, which are used throughout the books in this series, are indicated by a coloured corner flash to distinguish them from the rest of the text.

Introduction

Mental Disorder is a generic term. As defined in the Mental Health Act 1983 it covers:

(a) Mental illness.
(b) Psychopathic disorder.
(c) Mental handicap.
(d) Severe mental handicap.

This book has been written specifically for the nursing student in general training, who is gaining experience in the care and welfare of the mentally ill. It aims to give the nursing student both an insight into the problems experienced by people who are mentally ill, and into the role of the nurse in promoting the patient's recovery. Furthermore it aims to facilitate the learner's adjustment from the general hospital environment to the very different milieu of the psychiatric hospital.

The psychiatric nurse, and the nursing student in general training, is concerned with the promotion of mental health, the prevention of mental ill health, as well as caring for the person who has a mental disorder.

The aim of the experience in the care and welfare of the mentally ill in the general training programme is to enable the nursing student to develop further her skills in interpersonal relationships, her observation and communication skills and her ability to empathise. In particular, the emphasis will be on the development of non-verbal skills. During this experience the nursing student will spend the majority of her time sharing the daily living activities with her patients/clients. This means she will be doing less *for* them, and sharing more *with* them than she has been used to in general nursing. As a result she may find her role more emotionally demanding, with less heavy, physical work. She may feel vulnerable without the protection of a uniform if this is the policy in the unit. She will play and work with her patients, being sensitive to changes in tension levels, and alert to any indication of changing needs or behaviour. During this experience she will be able to gain an insight into the problems experienced by the mentally ill person, and of the role of the psychiatric *nurse* and other team members who work together to promote recovery and the mental health of patients and clients.

It is often difficult to differentiate between physical and mental illness, because of the interrelationship between mind and body, disturbance of the one affecting the other. Clare[1] suggests 'the concept of mental illness appears to permit a bewildering number of interpretations'. In mental illness there may be disturbance of the individual's personality, evidenced by the behaviour produced, which may prevent the person from carrying out his normal functions, and interferes with his interpersonal relationships. The mentally ill person can appear to behave quite normally on casual acquaintanceship, and it is only when the nursing student gets to know him well that his behaviour may appear unusual, deviating from his normal pattern. The nursing student may also find that the patient's behaviour is less predictable when he is mentally ill.

The treatment and care of the mentally ill person has changed over the years. In part this reflects the changing methods used to treat the mentally ill. Custodial care in large isolated asylums has been replaced by care in the person's home, or in psychiatric units in general hospitals, in hostels and day units, as well as in psychiatric hospitals.

Custodial care has given way to dynamic therapies and treatments carried out by the health care team, of which the patient is an active participant, and the psychiatric nurse an important member.

The emergence of treatments such as the major tranquilliser drugs has meant that the sick person can be cured, or his symptoms may be controlled sufficiently so that he can take his place in society.

Causes of mental illness

Mental illness results from a number of factors, some intrinsic, others external to the individual; sometimes the cause is multifactoral, affecting anyone regardless of age, sex, culture, race and social class.

Heredity, organic disease, biochemical disturbances, social and cultural pressures, disturbances in family relationships as well as age, sex, race and social class are all thought to be involved.

(a) Heredity

There is some evidence to suggest that some types of illness may be inherited. For example, some forms of schizophrenia. Twin studies suggest that the concordance rate in identical twins is about 40 per cent. In non-identical twins it is about 10 per cent and is higher if they are the same sex[2]. Huntington's Chorea is an example of a mental illness which is genetically determined.

(b) Organic disorders

Disturbance of brain cell function can be caused by an excess of alcohol and other poisons, drug intakes, brain tumour or head injury, or infection, or by a lack of oxygen, or an imbalance of fluid and electrolytes. Sometimes the cause is not known.

Cerebral arteries can become hardened and narrowed by the deposit of fatty plaques in the walls *(atheroma)* interfering with the blood supply. The function of the brain cells is disturbed, and if the cause is not found and rectified, eventually they die giving rise to the features of *organic brain syndrome* or *dementia*.

(c) Biochemical disturbances

It is generally accepted that some mental illness may in part be due to a disturbance in body chemistry. Depression, for example, can follow childbirth, or accompany the menopause, when the hormone levels are disturbed.

It is sometimes difficult to assess if the depression is caused by the changes in the hormone levels in the blood, or if the person is depressed because of a reaction to childbirth, or to the menopause. It is certainly the case that quite severe depressive illnesses can be triggered off by physical illness, for example, influenza, glandular fever, minor head injury with no significant organic cerebral damage.

Certain individuals with depressive illness have been found to have some deficiency of a particular substance in the brain *(serotonin)*.

Disturbance of sodium and water is thought to be a factor in the causation of mental illness where the mood is particularly affected *(mania, depression)*.

Drugs to remedy biochemical disturbances are given as a part of the total treatment of the individual.

(d) Social pressures

Many individuals cope with the stresses of everyday life, others cope with help, while others may become mentally ill.

Someone who has lost a dearly loved friend or relative should be allowed to work through their grief in their own way. If this is prevented, or if the person cannot cope with his feelings, he may become mentally ill, for example *depressed*.

(e) Family relationships

Relationships developed in the early formative years help the child 'pattern' his responses to others in later years. The child shown he is loved will probably grow up secure in his handling of relationships. Sometimes other members of the family blame a particular child for all the problems which arise in their family group, in other words the child becomes a *scapegoat* and if he cannot cope may withdraw into his own fantasy world, to such a degree that he may exhibit very disturbed behaviour.

A child may become confused by his mother continually saying she loves him but never demonstrating this by cuddling, kissing or touching. The child is in a double-blind situation and is so distressed that he becomes ill.

(f) Age

Some illnesses are more common at a particular age, e.g. organic brain syndrome in the elderly.

There are periods in the life pattern when an individual is more vulnerable to mental illness, for example on retirement from work, 'reactive' depression may occur.

(g) Sex

Admission rates of patients to hospital for affective disorders, e.g. depression, usually show a proportion of three females to two males.

(h) Race

Some races appear to be more prone to a particular mental illness, for example manic depressive disorder is said to be more common among members of the Jewish race.

(i) Social class

Certain forms of mental illness appear more commonly in certain social class groupings. For example, schizophrenia is more common in people working in semi-skilled or unskilled occupations (social classes IV and V on the Registrar General's Classification). It is suggested, however, that the very nature of this illness itself causes the individual to drift downward in the social scale[3].

Classification of mental illness

There are many ways of classifying mental illness, and it is important to remember that classifications are for ease of reference, and that nothing is absolute. There are no set patterns of behaviour for a specific illness, because an individual may respond in his own particular way.

Many books on psychiatry divide mental illnesses into the *neuroses* and *psychoses*. The term neurosis, sometimes referred to as psychoneurosis, means that the individual is normally aware he has a problem and has some understanding or insight about himself and the way he is reacting. The term psychosis usually refers to an illness in which the patient is out of touch with reality in the acute phase, appearing to withdraw into his own world. This is sometimes called an acute psychotic state.

It is often convenient to classify the mental illnesses according to the predominant features exhibited by the individual, as follows.

(a) Disorders of mood and emotion (the term *affect* is often used instead of mood)

A person who is depressed, or in the manic phase of the illness, is said to have an affective disorder. In the depressive stage the mood may range from sadness to despair, while in mania the mood may appear to be one of elation.

(b) Disorders of perception

Misinterpretation of a stimulus is known as an *illusion*. An example is the old lady shouting with fear that someone is coming through the window when it is the curtain moving. This can occur in health, as in the situation when an individual is in a highly anxious state, e.g. walking in the dark in strange surroundings, and is sometimes more pronounced in an illness like organic brain syndrome.

Hallucinations occur without an external stimulus, arising internally within the individual's thought processes and projected as real, and any of the five senses may be affected. For example, a person may see and hear people who are not there or he may feel, smell or taste objects which are not real. In schizophrenia, for example, auditory hallucinations are common.

(c) Disorders of thinking

Thought processes can sometimes be slowed, or retarded, which may happen in depression, or they may be speeded up, as in mania, where there is a continual flow of speech with topics changed frequently (a flight of ideas).

A *delusion* is a false fixed fact or belief held by a person, and can arise from an attempt by the individual to rationalise abnormal feelings, thoughts or actions.

There are different types of delusion. For example, an individual may believe he is Napoleon, and behave appropriately to his belief; this is a grandiose delusion, as may occur in mania.

(d) Disorders of memory

Some elderly patients find it relatively easy to recall incidents or events which happened when they were young, but cannot remember the way to the lavatory which was shown to them that morning. This can occur in organic brain syndrome, but as the illness progresses loss of memory extends increasingly so that early events are not recalled.

(e) Disorders of intellect

A person may be disorientated, that is, not know where he is, who he is, or the month of the year. This can occur in *acute confusional states,* such as in a person who has taken a drug overdose, or in an acute infectious illness. A state of progressive intellectual impairment occurs in organic brain syndrome, and the memory is also affected.

(f) Disorders of movement

A person may go through a set sequence of movements, for example, a ritual when washing hands. This can occur in *obsessional compulsive states.* In this illness the person knows his actions are illogical but is compelled to carry out the actions.

Further reading

Altschul, A., *Psychiatric Nursing,* 5th edn, Baillière Tindall, 1977

Carr, P.J., Butterworth, C.A. and Hodges, B.E., *Community Psychiatric Nursing,* Churchill Livingstone, 1980

Trethowan, W.H., *Psychiatry,* 4th edn, Baillière Tindall, 1979

Dally, P. and Harrington, H., *Psychology and Psychiatry for Nurses,* Hodder and Stoughton, reprinted 1977

Stuart, G.W. and Sundeen, S.J., *Principles and Practice of Psychiatric Nursing,* Mosby, 1979

Clare, A., *Psychiatry in Dissent,* 2nd edn, Tavistock Publications, 1980

Green, H., *I Never Promised You a Rose Garden,* Pan Books, 13th printing, 1982

Curran, D., Partridge, M. and Storey, P., *Psychological Medicine: An Introduction to Psychiatry,* 8th edn, Churchill Livingstone, 1976

References

1. Clare, A., *Psychiatry in Dissent: Controversial Issues in Thought and Practice,* 2nd edn, Tavistock Publications, 1980
2. Curran, D., Partridge, M. and Storey, P., *Psychological Medicine: An Introduction to Psychiatry,* 8th edn, Churchill Livingstone, 1976
3. Trethowan, W.H., *Psychiatry,* 4th edn, Baillière Tindall, 1979

Models in nursing

In the United Kingdom, interest in nursing models has been growing for a number of years. Perhaps it is unfortunate that the nursing process has been widely adopted before nurses have had the opportunity to learn about nursing models. A model is a representation of something but is not the real thing. For example, a model or diagram of the heart *represents* the heart, but it is *not* the heart. A nursing model can provide a framework of related concepts or ideas on which to base nursing practice. Some models provide parameters for patient assessment (see Collins and Parker: *Essentials of Nursing: An Introduction,* Chapter 1).

As the use of nursing models is relatively new in this country, research is needed to measure whether their use makes any substantial difference to the effectiveness of care. For more information on nursing models readers are referred to the suggested reading list at the end of this chapter.

Two models for psychiatric nursing

(a) Peplau's developmental model

Peplau's[4] Developmental Model has served as a conceptual framework for psychodynamic nursing since the publication of her book *Interpersonal Relations in Nursing* in 1952. Her model is based on four assumptions:

- Man is an organism living in an unstable environment. He has the ability to learn, to develop skills for problem-solving and to adapt to the tension created by needs.
- The kind of person each nurse becomes makes a substantial difference to what each patient will learn.
- The fostering of personality growth in the direction of position behaviour is the function of nursing and nursing education.
- The nursing profession has a legal responsibility for the effective use of nursing and its consequences for patients.

Peplau considers nursing as a 'significant therapeutic, interpersonal process'. The interpersonal process is central to her model and based on the active involvent of both the nurse and the patient. Personal growth and maturation are the focus of the interpersonal process for *both* participants. The process moves through four distinct phases, although some overlapping occurs.

Phase 1: Orientation

At the beginning of this phase the nurse and patient meet as strangers and the nurse offers the same courtesies that would be offered to a guest in a new situation.

The nurse helps the patient and/or his family to become aware of her availability to participate effectively in his health care. The orientation phase allows time for trust to develop. Learning may take place during this phase for the patient, but the nurse *must* learn while proceeding with an attitude of professional closeness. Peplau emphasises the difference between friendship and the nurse–patient relationship which exists primarily because of the needs of the patient.

Phase 2: Identification

The second phase of the interpersonal process allows the nurse to facilitate the expression of needs and problems by the patient. Stressful situations for the patient are identified through therapeutic conversation.

Phase 3: Exploitation

This is the working phase of the model in which the patient is able to derive full benefit from the relationship. The nurse utilises knowledge and skills derived from research and awareness of self. Other professional services are used if necessary.

In practice this phase takes the greatest amount of time to complete. The nurse intervenes with a wide repertoire of communication skills which help the patient to view his problems realistically and work towards anxiety reduction (Collister[1]). Maturation is the goal for both participants in the interaction.

Phase 4: Resolution

This is the final phase of the interpersonal process in which the nurse–patient relationship is terminated. Dependence is relinquished and the patient resumes independence. The nurse evaluates the personal growth that has occurred in both people, that is the patient *and* the nurse. Resolution of the nurse–patient relationship may be difficult for each or both parties if dependence needs are not relinquished.

Throughout the different phases of the interpersonal process the nurse adopts a number of different roles. These roles are adopted in accordance with the patient's situation experience and level of interaction and they include the following.

Resource Person

The nurse provides specific information to aid the patient's understanding of underlying problems. The nature of the patient's problems may necessitate referral to other professionals with appropriate expertise.

Teacher

The nurse imparts knowledge in accordance with the patient's needs and interests. Peplau[5] stresses the importance of being creative and using experiential learning as an educative instrument.

Leader

The nurse acts as a democratic leader by encouraging participation.

Surrogate

The nurse may take the place of another, e.g. mother, father, sibling, in situations that require the resolution of past or present interpersonal conflicts.

Counsellor

This role enables the nurse to communicate with the patient therapeutically and promote effective health-seeking outcomes.

Stranger

The nurse and patient meet as strangers and the nurse should convey the same courtesies that would be offered to a guest who was brought into a new situation.

Peplau		Nursing Process
Nurse and Patient		*Nurse and Patient*
Orientation	–	Assessment
Identification	–	Planning
Exploitation	–	Implementation
Resolution	–	Evaluation

Figure 0.1 Peplau's four phases have similarities with the nursing process

While Peplau's model has been criticised for its lack of structure (Heyman and Shaw[2]) it relates a limited number of concepts in an understandable way and provides clear direction for nursing practice. The model provides a useful framework for psychiatric nursing and for any nursing situation in which a nurse is engaged in a therapeutic relationship with a patient (Reed and Johnson[8]). Psychiatric nursing is carried out in an informal setting in which flexible approaches must be used to meet the needs of individual patients.

Iveson-Iveson[3] compared the phases of Peplau's Model with the stages of the nursing process (see Figure 0.1). This integration is further demonstrated by Pocock[7] and is particularly relevant to the practice of psychiatric nursing (Figure 0.2).

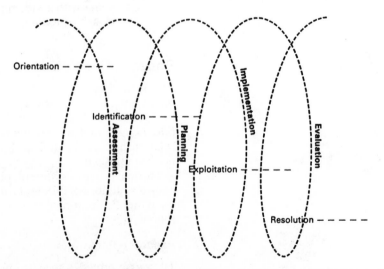

Figure 0.2 The similarities between phases of the nurse–patient relationship and the nursing process. (From an idea by Peter Pocock[7] and used with his permission)

References

1. Collister, B., Psychiatric nursing and a developmental model. In: Kershaw B. and Salvage J. (Eds), *Models for Nursing*, Wiley, 1986
2. Heyman B. and Shaw M., Looking at relationships in nursing. In: Skevington S. (Ed.), *Understanding Nurses*, Wiley, 1984
3. Iveson-Iveson, J., A two way process, *Nursing Mirror*, **155** (18), 52, 1982
4. Peplau, Hildegard E., *Interpersonal Relations in Nursing*, G. P. Putnam's Sons, New York, 1952
5. Peplau, H. E., What is experiential teaching? *American Journal of Nursing*, **57** (7), 884–886, 1957
6. Peplau, H. E., Interpersonal techniques: the crux of psychiatric nursing. In Smoyak S.A., and Rouslin S. (Eds), *A Collection of Classics in Psychiatric Nursing Literature*, Charles B. Slack, New Jersey, 1982
7. Pocock, P., Personal communication, 1986
8. Reed P. G. and Johnson, R. L., Peplau's nursing model: the interpersonal process. In: Fitzpatrick J. and Whall A. (Eds), *Conceptual Models of Nursing*: *Analysis and Application*, Rober J. Brady, Bowie, Maryland, 1983

(b) A philosophy and science of caring

Watson's[2] conceptual framework for nursing practice is based on a science of caring. She believes that nursing must achieve a delicate balance between scientific knowledge and the practice of humanistic caring behaviours. Nurses are concerned with the promotion of health, the prevention of illness, care of the sick and the restoration of health. Effective caring promotes health and growth. While caring (and nursing) exists in every society, caring attitudes are not transmitted genetically. Watson suggests that caring is a universal social phenomenon that can only be practised on an interpersonal basis.

Nursing has always been associated with caring in relation to other human beings, but this stance has been threatened by a long history of procedure-orientated nursing and discrepancies between theory and practice on the scientific and artistic aspects of caring. Watson strongly believes that opportunities for nurses to obtain advanced education will allow nursing to combine its caring humanistic orientation with relevant science.

Ten *carative factors* form the conceptual framework for understanding nursing as a science of caring. These carative factors are:

1. The formation of a humanistic-altruistic system of values.
2. The instillation of faith-hope.
3. The cultivation of sensitivity to one's self and to others.
4. The development of a helping-trusting relationship.
5. The promotion and acceptance of the expression of positive and negative feelings.
6. The systematic use of the scientific problem-solving method for decision-making.
7. The promotion of interpersonal teaching-learning.
8. The provision of a supportive, protective, and/or corrective mental, physical, sociocultural and spiritual environment.
9. Assistance with the gratification of human needs.
10. The allowance for existential-phenomenological forces.

The first three carative factors are interrelated and form a philosophical foundation for the science of caring.

1 Formation of a humanistic-altruistic value system

Watson argues that caring must be grounded on a set of universal human values and there must be a 'commitment to and satisfaction of receiving through giving'. Having a humanistic altruistic value system does not mean that the nurse has to be self-sacrificing or self-denying, it means that the self should be developed in a humanizing way and that the nurse should be aware of this sense of self.

2 Instillation of faith-hope

The second carative factor interacts with the humanistic altruistic value system to enhance other carative factors. The nurse must not ignore the role of faith and hope in carative and curative processes, and must recognise the importance of mental processes in the power of suggestion and placebo effects and the power of the relationship. The healing power of belief should not be overlooked in determining outcomes.

3 The cultivation of sensitivity to one's self and others

Sensitivity to one's self may determine the extent to which the nurse is able to develop the self and utilise the self with others. Watson[2] argues that too often people allow themselves to think their thoughts rather than to feel them and that nurses frequently hide behind impersonal, detached professional relationships in which feelings are hidden in a way that can be detrimental to the nurse-patient relationship. She suggests that many people fail to achieve their potential for development because they tend to look for opportunities outside themselves when the source for development is from within. She emphasises the need for nurses to be genuine to themselves and their feelings: 'Honesty towards self promotes authenticity and sensitivity towards others and it lays a foundation for primary prevention'. The nurse who is sensitive to the feelings of another person is able to make him feel understood, accepted and capable of moving towards mature levels of growth and functioning.

4 Development of a helping-trusting relationship

The development of a helping-trusting relationship is based on the previous carative factors. Watson emphasises that it is the *quality* of a person's relationship with another person that is significant in determining the *effectiveness* of helping behaviours.

Trust is basic to the relationship and essential for promoting personal and social growth and developing health-seeking behaviours. The nurse's sensitivity in interpersonal communication is one of the most crucial therapeutic tools for the delivery of care.

5 Promotion and acceptance of the expression of positive and negative feelings

This is an inherent part of the helping relationship. The expression of feelings is important, because feelings have a powerful effect on behaviour. The expression of strong negative feelings can allow a person to interact more freely, and to discover parts of himself of which he was previously unaware. The nurse must be supportive enough to permit such risk taking in the self as well as in others. Another person's feelings of fear or anger must be accepted without discomfort.

6 The systematic use of the scientific problem-solving method for decision-making

Watson argues that the nursing process and the scientific methods are basically the same and just as important as the humanistic approach to nursing. If nursing care is carried out without the scientific problem-solving method then she suggests 'effective practice is accidental at best and haphazard or harmful at worst'.

7 The promotion of interpersonal teaching-learning

Health teaching is one of the nurse's main functions and she or he must assess what the person needs to know in relation to present stresses. The giving of information can reduce a person's emotional response to stressful procedures that are often necessary in the overall treatment plan, e.g. injections, diagnostic examinations and treatment procedures. Watson emphasises the importance of patient learning that can have a balancing effect on behaviour and restore the person's state of equilibrium.

8 Provision for a supportive protective and/or corrective mental, physical, sociocultural and spiritual environment

A number of complex factors interact in the implementation of effective caring. The interdependence of internal and external environment is known to influence health and any change in a person's external or internal environment can lead to a stress change which a person will attempt to cope with. Watson describes four factors which can provide support for a person's internal and external environments.

Comfort

Comfort activities can provide support, protection and even correction. In providing comfort the nurse should help the person to function as effectively as possible, bearing in mind that intervention should be aimed at promoting health and independence.

Privacy

Hospitalisation can lead to a person's loss of privacy and subsequent de-personalisation. Professional integrity and confidentiality are integral parts of privacy concerns for the nurse. Privacy has a number of functions; it gives emotional release from the stresses of daily life; it gives a person time to integrate their feelings and experience; and it excludes others from certain knowledge about one's self.

Safety

This is crucial in caring for a person who is ill, excited, anxious or experiencing loss of control of their environment. Providing safety is basic to the nurse's role and affects activities in which the nurse supports, protects or corrects the environment.

Clean, aesthetic surroundings

Most people appreciate surroundings which are clean, aesthetic and at the same time, personalised. A person's health can be improved by pleasant surroundings. A person's self-concept and self-worth can be strengthened by the aesthetics of their environment.

9 Assistance with the gratification of human needs

Assistance with the gratification of human needs is basic to caring. Lower order needs incorporate those for survival and include the need for food and fluid, elimination and ventilation. Functional needs cover the need for activity and inactivity and the need for sexuality. Integrative needs embody the needs for achievement and affiliation while the highest order need is for self-actualisation which includes the growth-seeking need province.

10 The allowance for existential-phenomenological forces

This final carative factor acknowledges the personal subjective experience of a person as a foundation for understanding. Phenomenology is directed towards descriptions of what a person has come to know and understand in his experience: 'Existential experience infers a human awareness of the self and of otherness. It calls for a recognition of each man as existing singularly in his situation and struggling and striving with his fellows for survival and becoming, for confirmation of his existence and understanding of its meaning' (Paterson and Zderad[1]).

1. Paterson, J. G. and Zderad, L. T., *Humanistic Nursing*, Wiley, 1976
2. Watson, Jean, *Nursing. The Philosophy and Science of Caring*, Little, Brown and Co., Boston, 1979

The Nursing process

The nursing process is a systematic approach to patient care. Each patient's needs or problems are identified, nursing care is planned, implemented, and the effectiveness of care evaluated. The nursing process consists of four ongoing stages:

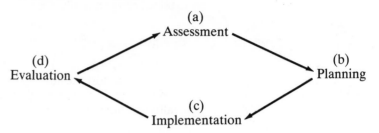

(a) Assessment

Assessment is the initial stage in which the nurse collects information about the patient, either from the patient himself or from his relatives or significant others.

The information is gained not only from verbal statements but also from observation of what the patient is saying through his body language. The information is recorded on a nursing history sheet. The design of data collection sheets varies between and sometimes within Health Authorities. Information is also obtained from documentation and members of other disciplines.

When carrying out an initial interview with a patient it is most important to focus on the patient as a person and not on the assessment form. In other words the nursing interview must not be allowed to become a mere paper exercise. In psychiatric nursing a person will only reveal things about himself as he begins to know and trust the nurse, therefore, the initial interview may be postponed so that some degree of trust may be established. Assessment is ongoing activity and the nurse will learn much about the patient and his problems during daily interactions.

The nurse–patient relationship is the key factor in all stages of the nursing process and requires the development of high-level interpersonal skills. The nurse who is able to get to know the patient really well will learn to understand his problems and needs from his own point of view.

(b) Planning

Whenever possible the nurse should work with the patient and his family in formulating a plan of care. Patient goals are stated for each of the identified needs or problems and nursing goals are clearly stated in order of priority to give clear directions for nursing interventions. The plan must state the nature of the nursing interventions so that nurses are able to focus their efforts towards the achievement of specific goals. The planning of nursing care cannot take place in isolation and must take into consideration the goals of other members of the multidisciplinary team.

(c) Implementation

Implementation refers to the actual giving of nursing care. Nursing interventions should be guided by the nursing care plan so that each nurse can be very clear in his or her own mind about the appropriate nursing behaviours. For example, a patient may need a sympathetic ear to listen to his feelings about his wife's death. The nursing orders in his plan of care may state 'Listen actively'. The nurse will know that active listening requires responses that enable the patient to know that he is being heard. These responses will primarily focus on the use of body language and will include eye contact, questions, head nods, facial expression and posture. Although each nurse will be directed through the nursing care plan to use the same interventions, each will bring his or her own unique interpretation to the nursing situation based on personality, experience and the level of self-awareness achieved.

(d) Evaluation

Evaluation is the fourth stage in the nursing process, in which the achievement of both patient and nursing goals is determined.

Evaluation may occur at the following times:

1. Some evaluation will be on-going and take place during and after a nursing procedure or intervention. This kind of evaluation is an integral and important part of the nursing process, as it enables the nurse to modify the care plan immediately in response to the patient's changing problems.

2. Other kinds of evaluation will occur on predetermined dates which have been set aside to evaluate the patient's goal achievement in relation to particular problems. This allows the nurse and patient to monitor progress.

3. Periodically there may be an evaluation of the overall nursing plan, in which problem statements, goals and nursing interventions will be placed under close scrutiny. The patient's goals may be examined to see if they were realistic and achievable and reflected the patient's problems adequately. The nursing orders may be studied to see if sufficient direction was given to the nursing interventions and the nursing interventions may be examined to see if they were appropriate and effective in helping the patient to achieve his goals.

The evaluation of each stage of the nursing process allows the nurse to review performance and aim towards quality care.

Suggested Reading

Aggleton P. and Chalmers H., Models and theories. 7. Henderson's Model, *Nursing Times*, **81** (10), 33–35, 1985

Aggleton P. and Chalmers H., Models and theories. 5. Orem's self-care model, *Nursing Times*, **81** (1), 36–39, 1985

Aggleton P. and Chalmers H., Models and theories. 2. The Roy adaptation model, *Nursing Times*, **80** (40), 45–48, 1984

Aggleton P. and Chalmers H., Models and theories. 3. The Riehl interaction model, *Nursing Times*, **80** (45), 58–61, 1984

Aggleton P. and Chalmers, H., *Nursing Models and the Nursing Process*, Macmillan Education, 1986

Arumugan, U., Helping Harry to relate to others. *Nursing Times*, **81** (21), 43–45, 1985 (uses Riehl model)

Barker J., A plan for Arthur and Mary, *Nursing Times*, Community outlook, November 14th, 1984 (uses Orem model)

Hardy L. K., Nursing models and research — a restricting view, *Journal of Advanced Nursing*, **7**, 447–451, 1982

Hoeffner B. and Murphy S., The unfinished task: development of nursing theory for psychiatric and mental health nursing practice, *Journal of Psychosocial Nursing and Mental Health Services*, **20** (12), 8–14, 1982

Hoon, E., Game playing: a way to look at nursing models, *Journal of Advanced Nursing*, **11**, 421–427, 1986

Iveson – Iveson J., A two-way process, *Nursing Mirror*, **155** (18), 52, 1982 (Peplau model)

Iveson – Iveson J., Putting ideas into action, *Nursing Mirror*, **155** (16), 49, 1982 (Orem Model)

McGlynn J., The quest for nursing knowledge, *Nurse Education Today*, **4** (2), 46–47, 1984

Moscovitz A. O., Orem's theory as applied to psychiatric nursing, *Perspectives in Psychiatric Care*, **22** (1), 36–38, 1984

O'Rawe A. M., Self neglect — a challenge for nursing, *Nursing Times*, **78** (46), 1932–1936, 1982 (uses Orem model)

O'Toole A. W., When the practical becomes theoretical, *Journal of Psychosocial Nursing and Mental Health Services*, **19** (12), 11–19, 1981

Pearson, A. and Vaughan, B., *Nursing Models for Practice*, Heinemann, 1986

Price B., Just a few forms to fill in, *Nursing Times*, **79** (44), 26–29, 1983

Runtz S. E. and Urtel, J. G., Evaluating your practice via a nursing model, *Nurse Practitioner*, **8** (3), 32 and 37–40, 1983 (two case examples using Orem and Peplau)

Stockwell F., *The Nursing Process in Psychiatric Nursing*, Croom Helm, 1985

Webb, C., Nursing models: A personal view, *Nursing Practice*, **1**, 208–212, 1986

Mental Health Act 1983
Some Common Sections

Section	Reasons	Duration	Action before expiration	Extension
Informal	Patient is not unwilling to be admitted to hospital without formality. Can discharge himself	—	—	—
2	Compulsory Admission for Assessment — can include compulsory treatment. Application made by nearest relative or Approved Social Worker, supported by two medical recommendations. Nearest relative can discharge patient. Patient can appeal to the Mental Health Review Tribunal (MHRT) in first 14 days.	28 days	(a) Discharge (b) Admit informally (c) Admit for treatment (Section 3)	—
3	Compulsory Treatment Order for mentally disordered & impaired & psychopathic patients if disorder is of a nature & degree that warrants treatment & is likely to benefit. Application made by nearest relative or Approved Social Worker if nearest relative consents; or is displaced by County Court or is not reasonably practical to consult nearest relative. Approved Social Worker to provide social circumstances & report to hospital. Two medical recommendations — one approved — one knowing patient & not from same hospital unless delay would cause serious risk to health & safety of patient. Patient can apply to MHRT in first 6 months; second 6 months; then annually.	6 months	(a) Discharge (b) Admit informally (c) Renew S.3 Renewal can be authorised if patient is still mentally disordered & medical treatment in hospital is appropriate & cannot be given unless detention continues OR patient is unlikely to be able to care for self, obtain care needed or to guard self against exploitation.	6 months then annually
4	Compulsory Emergency Admission for Assessment. Application by nearest relative or Approved Social Worker who must have seen patient within previous 24 hours and patient must be admitted within 24 hours of completed application &/or medical recommendation.	72 hours	(a) Discharge (b) Admit informally (c) Convert to S.2 or 3 with 2nd. medical recommendation	—
5	Compulsory detention of informal patient seeking discharge who is a danger to self &/or others. Order signed by Dr in charge of treatment or another nominated hospital doctor. An RMN or RNMS can invoke holding power until Dr arrives if nurse considers patient's health/safety &/or protection of others warrants immediate restraint. Official record to be kept.	72 hours 6hours	(a) Discharge (b) Revert to informal (c) Admit S.2 or 3	—
7 Guardian-ship	Application by 2 Drs to Local Social Services Dept (usually) if this is in patient's welfare interests. The LA has to approve person appointed guardian, if not itself. This requires patient to live at specified place, attend for treatment/occupation/training & power to ensure a Dr, Social Worker or others to see patient at home. Patient has same rights as informal patient regarding consent to treatment provisions.	—	—	—
23	Discharge of a compulsorily detained patient (Sections 2, 3 or 4).	—	—	—
47	Transfer of mentally ill person from prison to detention in hospital.	Until earliest date of release with remission	—	—
136	Compulsory removal to a place of safety by a constable of a person in a public place who appears mentally ill, in the interests of the person or protection of others.	72 hours	(a) Discharge (b) Admit informally (c) Admit under S.2 or 3	—
37	Hospital Court Order, recommended by 2 Drs either that mental disorder warrants detention in hospital OR mental impairment/psychopathic disorder is such that mental hospital treatment would alleviate or prevent a deterioration in offender's condition. Can apply to MHRT once in second 6 months & annually thereafter.	—	—	—
41	Restricted Court Order for protection of public from serious harm. MHRT procedure as for S.37	—	—	—
35 Remand to hospital	For medical report by Crown or Magistrates' Court. Covers all 4 categories of mental disorders.	Up to 28 days	—	Renewable for up to 12 weeks
36 Remand for treatment	For mental illness and severe mental impairment only by Crown Court. Remand to hospital only where bail is not possible.	Up to 28 days	—	Not more than 12 weeks
38 Interim hospital order	For assessment of Hospital Order by Crown or Magistrates' Court.	12 weeks	—	Up to 6 months

NB: This is purely an outline and the reader is recommended to refer to the full text of the Mental Health Act 1983, published by H.M.S.O., 1983

The principal members of the psychiatric treatment team

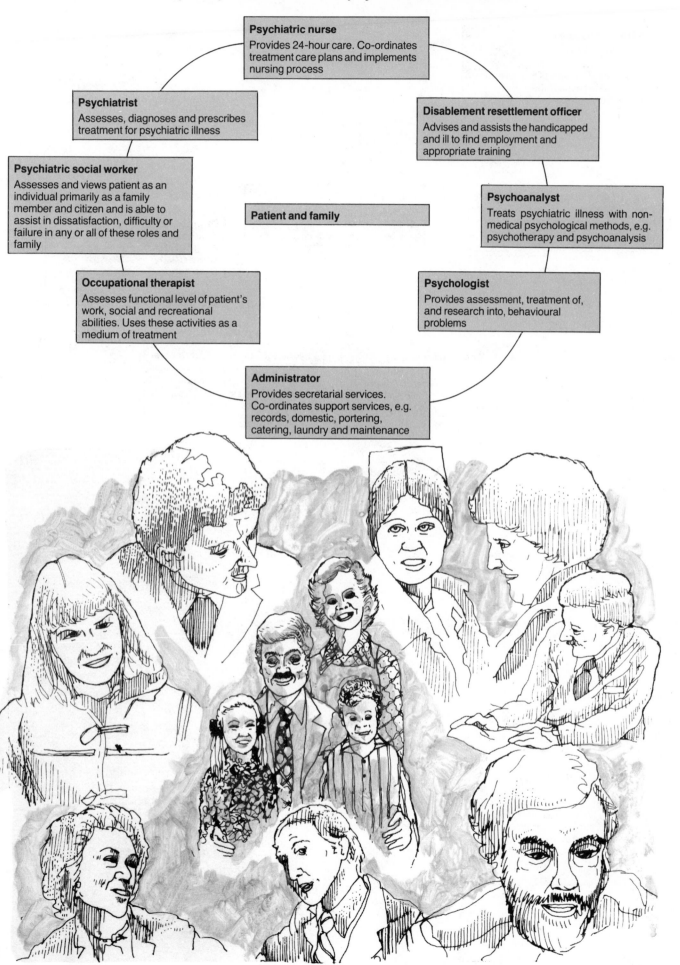

Psychiatric nurse
Provides 24-hour care. Co-ordinates treatment care plans and implements nursing process

Psychiatrist
Assesses, diagnoses and prescribes treatment for psychiatric illness

Disablement resettlement officer
Advises and assists the handicapped and ill to find employment and appropriate training

Psychiatric social worker
Assesses and views patient as an individual primarily as a family member and citizen and is able to assist in dissatisfaction, difficulty or failure in any or all of these roles and family

Patient and family

Psychoanalyst
Treats psychiatric illness with non-medical psychological methods, e.g. psychotherapy and psychoanalysis

Occupational therapist
Assesses functional level of patient's work, social and recreational abilities. Uses these activities as a medium of treatment

Psychologist
Provides assessment, treatment of, and research into, behavioural problems

Administrator
Provides secretarial services. Co-ordinates support services, e.g. records, domestic, portering, catering, laundry and maintenance

Various aspects of a comprehensive psychiatric service

Mental hospital
Has in-patient facilities. Many provide day- and out-patient facilities. The base of the main and support services of the comprehensive psychiatric service

Community psychiatric nursing service
Home nursing either as part of a comprehensive psychiatric service or of the primary health care team

Health centre
Psychiatrist and psychiatric nurse give counsel and treatment as members of primary team

Specialist units, e.g.:
Alcoholism Can offer in-, **Drug addiction** day- or out- **Children/** patient services. **adolescents** Often planned **Mother/baby** to serve a **Deaf/dumb** regional area **Therapeutic community**

Crisis intervention
Emergency psychiatric service, usually a doctor, nurse and social worker who will either visit crisis scene or have a 'walk-in' clinic

Psychiatric unit in District General Hospital
Has in-, out- and day-patient facilities, part of a total health service on one site and convenient to the community served

Sheltered workshops. Day centres. Clubs. Hostels. Half-way houses
Run by hospital, local authority or voluntary groups for discharged patients who need community help, support and supervision

Day hospital
Has facilities for treating patients who live in the community. Prevents institutionalisation

Out-patient clinic
Specialist treatment, assessment, advice. Often part of day hospital

Special hospital regional secure unit
In-patient facilities with high/medium security for mentally ill who have either committed a criminal act and been ordered there by court or cannot be managed in an open hospital. These serve a regional or larger area.

Various treatment models

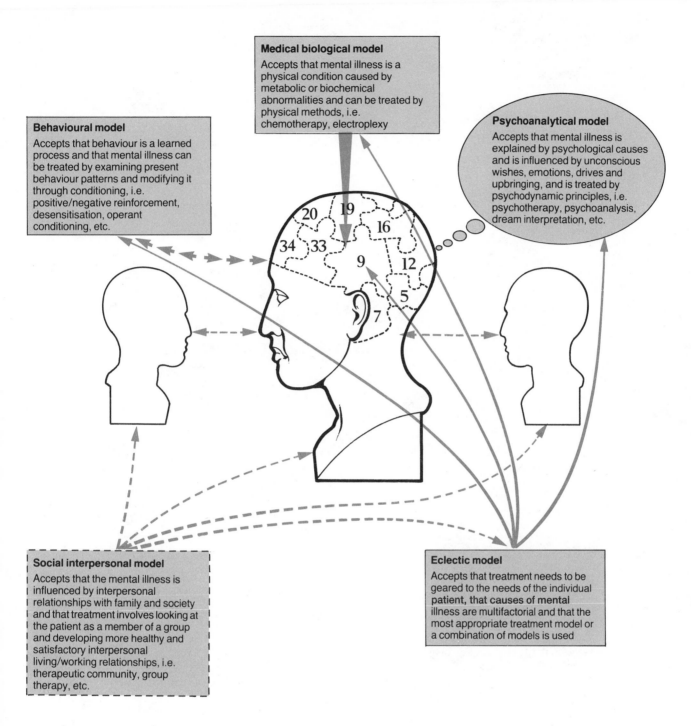

Medical biological model
Accepts that mental illness is a physical condition caused by metabolic or biochemical abnormalities and can be treated by physical methods, i.e. chemotherapy, electroplexy

Behavioural model
Accepts that behaviour is a learned process and that mental illness can be treated by examining present behaviour patterns and modifying it through conditioning, i.e. positive/negative reinforcement, desensitisation, operant conditioning, etc.

Psychoanalytical model
Accepts that mental illness is explained by psychological causes and is influenced by unconscious wishes, emotions, drives and upbringing, and is treated by psychodynamic principles, i.e. psychotherapy, psychoanalysis, dream interpretation, etc.

Social interpersonal model
Accepts that the mental illness is influenced by interpersonal relationships with family and society and that treatment involves looking at the patient as a member of a group and developing more healthy and satisfactory interpersonal living/working relationships, i.e. therapeutic community, group therapy, etc.

Eclectic model
Accepts that treatment needs to be geared to the needs of the individual patient, that causes of mental illness are multifactorial and that the most appropriate treatment model or a combination of models is used

Suggested reading

Jones, R. M., *The Mental Health Act*, Sweet and Maxwell, 1983

Chapter 1

Nursing the patient who is anxious

Introduction

Anxiety is the most universal of all human emotions. It is an energy that cannot be observed directly and must therefore be inferred from behaviour. Most people when faced with a new and unfamiliar situation will experience some degree of anxiety. Normal anxiety is proportional to the threat a person is faced with and can provide arousal that is appropriate to the situation. Mild levels of anxiety can be beneficial, acting as a motivating force, which enhances productivity and performance. Severe anxiety can have an inhibiting effect and move a person away from his optimal level of performance towards behaviours which are non-coping and maladaptive (Graves and Thompson[1]). The manifestations of anxiety are both physical and psychological (see Figure 1.1) and prepare the individual for fight or flight. While under normal circumstances changes in the functioning of the autonomic system heighten a person's capacity to deal with threats, severe anxiety can severely inhibit a person's level of functioning in so much that the ability to perceive accurately and without distortion is narrowed. In panic, the most extreme manifestation of anxiety, there is a total lack of focus and the person may thrash about purposelessly, his attention being unfocused and unchannelled in such a way that his safety may be threatened.

Psychological symptoms	Physical symptoms
Apprehension	Tremor
Tension	Sweating
Irritability	Dryness of mouth
Poor concentration	Dilated pupils
Insomnia	Tachycardia
Headaches	
Fatigue	
Dizziness	

Source: Harrison, R. J., *Textbook of Medicine with Relevant Physiology and Anatomy*, Hodder and Stoughton, London, 1977

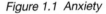

Figure 1.1 Anxiety

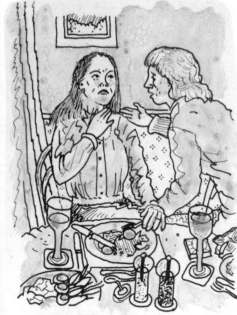

Under normal circumstances anxiety dimishes once a threat is removed; when anxiety becomes the focus of a person's daily living and is not evoked by any particular circumstances it is referred to as free floating anxiety.

The nursing care for the patient in the following profile is organised through the use of two separate nursing models in order to illustrate the application of two different frameworks for care. The first model is Peplau's[4] Developmental Model and the second is Watson's[8] Philosophy and Science of Caring in which Rebecca's care is planned using ten carative factors. (An overview of both models is given in the Introduction.)

Patient Profile

Rebecca Rawlings, aged 26, had been very concerned about her health for some months, and frequently visited her GP for reassurance. Rebecca found it difficult to put her feelings into words. She felt tense and 'on edge' all the time and had a vague sense of dread that something terrible was going to happen to her.

She avoided company because she felt ill at ease; she was unable to get her breath and had a fear of suffocation. Equally, she felt apprehensive when alone and was troubled by her pounding heart and profuse sweating. The unpleasant feelings had forced Rebecca to give up the voluntary work which she did with handicapped children. At her father's suggestion, since leaving school, Rebecca had been helping with the family business.

Dr Ludlow referred Rebecca to Glenys Brown, the Community Psychiatric Nurse.

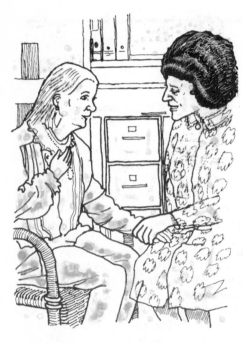

A plan of care using Peplau's Developmental Model

Having approached her doctor on numerous occasions Rebecca was only too willing to accept the help of the Community Psychiatric Nurse. The nurse decided to use Peplau's (1952) Developmental Model for Rebecca's care (see page 5).

As a prerequisite to helping Rebecca the nurse had to ask herself if her desire to help Rebecca was based on a sincere wish to help her in her present predicament, as insincerity would only add to the patient's burden by increasing her feelings of anxiety (Topalis and Aguilera[7]). For some nurses 'neurotic' behaviours can evoke negative feelings; because the patient's symptoms are emotionally caused there may be a tendency to discount their credibility (Macilwaine[3], Irving[2]).

(a) Orientation

During the Orientation phase the nurse conveyed her willingness to listen to Rebecca's problems (role of counsellor) and acted as a person who was willing to be receptive to her feelings (role of surrogate). Rebecca seemed to lack any confidence in herself and it was important for the nurse to make her feel accepted as a worthwhile human being. As the nurse worked towards establishing a nurse-patient relationship she helped Rebecca to understand the purpose of the relationship.

Rebecca saw her problems in physical terms and found it difficult to associate her present feelings with anxiety. While encouraging Rebecca to share her feelings the nurse avoided reinforcing physical complaints. As the relationship developed Rebecca began to accept the nurse as a trusted person. The nurse was able to give her an explanation (role of teacher) as to the relationship between mind and body. This information was given in a simple and concise way, bearing in mind that anxiety can inhibit a person's ability to 'hear'.

(b) Identification

Rebecca told the nurse that she had never experienced such terrible feelings in her life and thought that she was going to die. She felt out of control and at times she did not know what she was doing. The nurse was able to assess that the anxiety Rebecca was experiencing was both disabling and posed a threat to her safety. Her task was to help Rebecca recognise and resolve underlying problems that could be acting as stressors, by harnessing energies derived from anxiety and tension into productive energy for problem solving.

The nurse encouraged Rebecca to be open about her feelings without making any demands on her. Within the privacy of her own home Rebecca was helped to release her emotions. She was able to decide what information she wished to share with the nurse herself.

Although the nurse initially adopted the role of leader, she relinquished this role as quickly as possible, encouraging Rebecca to be actively involved in decisions concerning her own care.

The following nursing plan was formulated:

Patient problem	Patient goal	Nursing goal
Anxious and apprehensive. Feels threat to security/safety.	To reduce maladaptive anxiety.	Teach Rebecca to initiate relaxation.
Physical discomfort particularly sweating. Heart beating quickly.	To achieve physical comfort.	Help her to feel physically comfortable and at ease.
Lack of knowledge concerning mind and body relationships.	To understand the association between mind and body.	Choose appropriate methodology to enable Rebecca to learn about her body.
Family does not provide environment for expression of feelings.	To express undisclosed feelings.	Promote expression of feelings through the nurse-patient relationship.
Poor self-image. Lack of confidence. Uncomfortable with self and in presence of others.	To view self more positively. To increase self-confidence.	Assist Rebecca to develop positive self-perception and confidence in the presence of others. For the nurse to develop greater self-understanding and interpersonal growth through the process of helping Rebecca.

(c) Exploitation

During the working phase, the nurse respected Rebecca's need for greater personal space, but when her non-verbal behaviour indicated that her feelings of anxiety were heightened the nurse's sensitivity enabled her to offer reassurance through the use of touch. It was important to help Rebecca to use her own skills to work through problems. The nurse approached the physiotherapist (role of resource person) for instruction in relaxation exercises so that she could in turn teach Rebecca to gain mastery over her symptoms and indeed over her own life (see Figure 1.2).

When a person is anxious breathing becomes quick and irregular and only takes place in the upper part of the lungs; the accent is always on inspiration. If a person overbreathes the pH of the blood increases, causing dizziness and other unpleasant sensations. Relaxed breathing, on the other hand, is slow and regular and involves the lower part of the lungs. Rebecca was instructed to initiate self-control through relaxation in situations where she felt anxious. Rebecca's shoulders were always tilted upwards in a stress position. Mitchell (1977) suggests that tense people suffering from undischarged stress adopt particular patterns of positioning in all their joints. This can become a vicious circle if not interrupted. Rebecca was taught to pull her shoulders in a downward direction towards her feet while breathing in slowly and deeply with the accent on expiration.

Reference

Mitchell, L., *Simple Relaxation, the Physiological Method for Easing Tension*. John Murray, 1977

Bibliography

Priest, R., *Anxiety and Depression. A Practical Guide to Recovery*, Martin Dunitz, 1983

Figure 1.2 Relaxation

Rebecca told the nurse that her family never talked about feelings; she could not recall either of her parents ever crying even over events that aroused feelings of emotion in most other people. Rebecca described her parents as being very kind, but she felt that she had always been expected to help in the family business rather than develop an independent career for herself. Rebecca told the nurse that she was faced with the dilemma of wanting to leave home and lead her own independent life, but she was afraid that this would hurt her parents' feelings. Sometimes she felt guilty just thinking about it but at the same time she felt a certain anger and resentment because it seemed that they took her for granted. She also felt that her parents never really wanted to listen to any point of view other than their own and when they listened to her they were not really hearing what she said.

Rebecca told the nurse that she had never had any one that she could really confide in before. She actually felt relieved to be able to unburden her feelings to someone who was prepared to listen actively. She felt more able to deal with her feelings rationally once they were out in the open and in this way the nurse was able to help Rebecca to redirect the energy which had been anxiety-bound into productive energy for problem solving (see Figure 1.3).

Severe anxiety – Energy – Non-productive illness behaviours

Mild anxiety   – Energy – Productive health-seeking behaviours

---

Figure 1.3 Redirection of energy

Creating a therapeutic climate in which Rebecca could express her thoughts and feelings required a high degree of nursing skill. The nurse had to convey to Rebecca a sense of acceptance and a feeling that she would not be judged if she expressed attitudes and values which differed from those of the nurse.

The nurse encouraged Rebecca to widen her horizons by developing interests outside the home and family business. As the nurse discovered Rebecca's interests, several possibilities were explored; she decided that she would like to join a pottery making class and it was suggested to Rebecca that she should initiate her own enquiries. Taylor[6] suggests that it can be helpful for the anxious person to be provided with the opportunity to succeed, as this helps to build self-esteem and confidence. The nurse also referred Rebecca to a self-help group.

(d) Resolution

As Rebecca's capacities for the control of anxiety increased and she became more confident in dealing with her own company and the company of others, the need for the nurse-patient relationship was reduced. Rebecca was aware from the very beginning that the relationship was goal-centred and would eventually be terminated. Rebecca was able to relinquish her dependence on the nurse as she gained strength through other supportive networks. In evaluating the growth which had occurred in both Rebecca and herself the nurse felt that Rebecca had achieved more self-awareness and coping behaviours. Through helping Rebecca the nurse felt that she had learned a great deal about herself and her own need to succeed. Only time will tell if Rebecca can achieve her long-term goals and establish a life of her own away from her parents.

An approach to care using Watson's (1979) philosophy and science of caring

Carative Factors	Assessment	Planning		Implementation	Evaluation
		Patient goal	Nursing goal		
1. *The formation of a humanistic-altruistic system of values.*	Poor self-esteem manifested in discomfort in presence of others and negative self-statements. *Patient problem* Makes negative self-statements. Not at ease with others, especially people outside the family.	To gain a more positive self-image. To develop the confidence to be at ease in social situations.	To help Rebecca believe in her own self-worth and abilities.	The nurse needed not only to feel that Rebecca was a worthwhile human being but also to convey this to her within a supportive humanistic orientation. By being empathic the nurse entered Rebecca's feelings and experiences through positive feedback and gradually helped her to view herself and her abilities in a more favourable light.	As the therapeutic depth of interaction with Rebecca increased she began to feel more confident and was able to verbalise the good things about herself. Her relationship with the nurse formed a foundation for more fulfilling relationships with others.
2. *The instillation of faith-hope.*	Focuses on physical complaints. Fears serious illness. *Patient problem* Has doubts about ability to overcome physical problems. Poor understanding of association between emotion and ill health.	To demonstrate verbally an understanding of the relationship of body and mind in anxiety.	To teach Rebecca to understand the relationship between psychological and physiological functioning. Promote faith and hope. Enable her to believe in herself.	It was important for the nurse to convey to Rebecca that she *could* overcome her problem. Through discussion and feedback the nurse facilitated Rebecca's understanding of the relationship between mind and body functioning. When appropriate, and if the nurse thought it would enhance Rebecca's learning, she disclosed information about her own life where faith and hope had helped to develop greater self-understanding.	As Rebecca developed a sense of control over her body she began to accept that her problems were not insurmountable. She was able to give feedback to the nurse concerning her understanding of anxiety and its physical manifestations.
3. *The cultivation of sensitivity to one's self and to others.*	Potential for greater self-understanding demonstrated through present symptomatology.	To gain greater self-awareness.	Help Rebecca to gain greater understanding and self-awareness by creating an environment in which self-disclosure can be accepted.	In helping Rebecca come to terms with her problems the nurse was sensitive to her own feelings and body language. She accepted Rebecca's symptoms as a legitimate expression of her underlying problems, but avoided reinforcing her physical complaints. Because the patient's symptoms are emotionally caused there may be a tendency for some nurses to discount their credibility. As the nurse-patient relationship developed Rebecca was able to disclose and explore personal feelings.	The development of self-awareness was a long-term goal, and while Rebecca has developed some insight into her own behaviour through self-disclosure, greater self-awareness is still something Rebecca must strive for within the supportive framework of self-help groups.

Carative Factors	Assessment	Planning		Implementation	Evaluation
		Patient goal	Nursing goal		
4. *The development of a helping-trusting relationship.*	Parents are kind but do not express or encourage the expression of emotion. Rebecca thinks (as her parents do) that it is a sign of weakness. Feels somewhat guilty about her present state. *Patient problem* Ineffective support systems. Feels guilty about feelings.	To develop coping behaviours within a supportive framework. To talk about feelings without a sense of guilt.	To achieve a helping-trusting relationship with Rebecca and to assist her to develop a supportive network through self-help agencies.	By being authentic and honest the nurse provided a supportive, protective and corrective milieu. The nurse was aware that insincerity would only leave Rebecca feeling uneasy as to what to expect, and would inhibit the development of trust. Trust was essential to enable Rebecca to talk about her feelings.	Rebecca gradually learned that the expression of feelings constituted a health-seeking behaviour. As her confidence increased the nurse encouraged her to consider joining a self-help group.
5. *The promotion and acceptance of the expression of positive and negative feelings.*	As feelings are not discussed within the family, Rebecca has no venue to express a whole range of emotions. *Patient problem* Possible unresolved conflicts and feelings.	To express positive and negative feelings in nurse's presence.	To create a climate of acceptance in which Rebecca can express feelings.	The nurse encouraged Rebecca to share feelings by making her feel sufficiently comfortable in the relationship to take risks in disclosing feelings and unpleasant conversations which may not have been previously expressed without fear of accusation or argument. This necessitated the acceptance of Rebecca's feelings in a non-judgemental way and the ability for the nurse to come to terms with her own feelings. The expression of unresolved conflicts is important as feelings related to these may act as an agenda in adult life (Watson[8]).	Rebecca was able to talk openly about her needs for independence. She felt her parents overlooked her needs for an independent existence by taking her for granted and expecting her to work in the family business.
6. *The systematic use of scientific problem-solving method of decision-making.*	Assess Rebecca's problems using the scientific problem-solving method. *Patient problems* See 1–5 and 7–10.	Plan specific goals for patient to reduce anxiety.	Provide planned nursing interventions to enable nursing practice to be controlled instead of haphazard.	Use appropriate interventions to reduce anxiety, by enabling patient to engage in problem-solving activities which will ultimately diminish maladaptive behaviours.	Evaluation of goal achievement was discussed with Rebecca. While most goals were achieved, she had not yet made her final bid for independence. Having gained more confidence and self-control she has developed the 'tools' to accomplish this in her own good time.

Carative Factors	Assessment	Planning		Implementation	Evaluation
		Patient goal	Nursing goal		
7. *The promotion of interpersonal teaching-learning*	Rebecca is lacking in knowledge about the cause and effect of symptoms. Copes with stress by withdrawing because she finds it very threatening. *Patient problem* Knowledge deficit in relation to symptomatology. Tension, inability to relax. Apprehensive about unknown situations.	To gain self-control in all situations by increase in knowledge and the development of coping behaviours.	Help Rebecca to reduce threat by increasing knowledge and self-control mechanisms.	Rebecca was given information to enhance her self-control in all situations. Firstly she was taught relaxation techniques using the Laura Mitchell method (see Figure 1.2). Through role play she was encouraged to increase her controllability in potentially threatening situations which she had identified with the nurse. Role play can provide a person with the opportunity to try out new behaviours in a positive and safe setting (Pope[5]). When role play situations relate to the problems of everyday life the patient can be afforded the opportunity to explore behavioural patterns and practise skills which will ultimately increase his autonomy and independence.	Rebecca was greatly helped by being able to initiate relaxation through enacting the threatening situation she had identified, she felt less apprehensive and more confident in her ability to cope. Rebecca was gradually helped to perceive stress not as a threat but as a challenge and growth experience.
8. *The provision of a supportive, protective and/or corrective mental, physical, sociocultural and spiritual environment*	Never very confident. Rebecca wants to strive out alone but perhaps also uses parents need of her to prolong dependence because she lacks confidence. *Patient problem* Needs to function more independently of parents, but leads a sheltered life with few friends of own age.	To develop independence and peer group support.	Help Rebecca to widen her social network to enable her to develop friendships.	Rebecca was helped by the nurse to focus on interests outside herself. It was suggested that she might consider evening classes; when she felt confident enough to join a pottery class, the nurse encouraged Rebecca to make her own application and arrangements, thus enhancing her goals for independence and control over her own environment.	Rebecca persevered with the pottery class. She has developed a friendship with a girl who lives locally and has spoken of their plans to go on holiday together in the summer.

Carative Factors	Assessment	Planning		Implementation	Evaluation
		Patient goal	*Nursing goal*		
9. *Assistance with the gratification of human needs.*	Survival and safety needs threatened and therefore inhibiting higher orders needs for achievement and self-actualisation. Physical discomfort, i.e. tension, sweating. *Patient problem* Survival and safety needs are threatened by lack of self-control. Physical discomfort caused by anxiety.	Reduction in perceived threats to survival and safety. To develop the ability and confidence to meet higher order needs. To achieve physical comfort.	Promote control mechanisms to enable Rebecca to meet higher needs and physical comfort.	Self-control was enhanced by teaching Rebecca to initiate relaxation. This was important because if her levels of anxiety reached a state of panic, her perception would be so unfocused as to constitute a serious danger to her safety. The nurse initially advised Rebecca to wear loose cotton clothing to enhance her physical comfort.	When Rebecca developed self-control she was able to focus on the achievement of higher order needs. For example, her needs for creativity were satisfied through meeting needs to increase her social network.
10. *The Allowance for existential-phenomeno-logical forces.*	Personal subjective experiences have included fears of dying, symptoma-tology and dilemma concerning dependence/ independence. *Patient problem* The need to be recognised as an individual with hopes and desires.	To be recognised for individuality.	Appreciate Rebecca's subjective experiences from her own point of view.	Understand Rebecca's experiences and the meaning these experiences have for her. Remember that these experiences are for her as much a part of her human experience as any external indicators of behaviour.	Rebecca was recognised for her individuality and subjective experiences.

References

1. Graves, H. H. and Thompson, E. A., Anxiety: a mental health vital sign. In: Longo D. C. and Williams, R. A., (Eds), *Clinical Practice in Psycho-social Nursing: Assessment and Intervention*, Appleton-Century-Crofts, New York 1978
2. Irving, S., *Basic Psychiatric Nursing*, 2nd edn, W. B. Saunders Co., 1978
3. Macilwaine, H., How nurses and neurotic patients view each other in general hospital psychiatric units, *Nursing Times*, **77** (27), 1158–1160, 1981
4. Peplau, Hildegard E., *Interpersonal Relations in Nursing*, G. P. Putnam's Sons, New York, 1952
5. Pope, B., *Social Skills Training for Psychiatric Nurses*, Harper and Row London, 1986
6. Taylor, C. M., *Mereness Essentials of Psychiatric Nursing*, 11th edn, C. V. Mosby, St. Louis, 1982
7. Topalis M. and Aguilera, D., *Psychiatric Nursing*, 7th edn, C. V. Mosby, St. Louis, 1978
8. Watson, Jean, *Nursing. The Philosophy and Science of Caring*, Little, Brown & Co., Boston, 1979

Bibliography

Gregg, D., Reassurance, *American Journal of Nursing*, **55**, 171–174, 1955
Longo, D. C. & Williams, R. A. (Eds), *Clinical Practice in Psychosocial Nursing: Assessment and Intervention*, Appleton-Century-Crofts, New York, 1978

ASSESSMENT INTERVIEW

Consultant _____ —

GP _____ Dr M Ludlow

Referred by _____

Date of referral _____ Date of admission _____

Short-stay ward _____

Medium-stay ward _____

Long-stay ward _____

Day hospital _____

Community Nursing Service _____

Surname Mr/Mrs/Miss _Rawlings_

Forenames _Rebecca Kathleen_

Address _17 Station Rd, Raylton_

Tel. No. _616 7211_

Name of next of kin _Parents: Mr and Mrs C. Rawlings_

Address _Same address_

Tel. No. _____

Name by which the patient likes to be addressed
Rebecca

Birthday _13.5.60_

DESCRIPTION OF THE PATIENT

Colour of eyes _Blue_ Hair colour _Light brown_

Height (m) _1.676_ Weight (kg) _64.5_

Distinguishing features
Nose slightly prominent

Present occupation/Occupational history
Helps in family business (timber store) doing mostly clerical work.

Hobbies and interests
Sewing, reading.
Helps at Harewood House, Wednesday afternoons - likes children. Has not been for past 2 months.

Family or persons of significance in patient's life
Parents

Persons expected to visit
Not relevant

Religion
—

Home conditions
Lives in large detached house in same road as family business.

Community services involved/referred

Name of person _Glenys Brown_

Status _Community Psychiatric Nurse_

Tel. No. _3330_

Whether contacted (and reason for contacting, if relevant
Yes. Through GP.

PSYCHIATRIC CONDITION

Previous psychiatric illness
_No._
Has always consulted GP with minor complaints.

Present psychiatric condition

General appearance
Posture - shoulders hunched up.

Behaviour _Edgy, cannot rest. Taps fingers and plays with rings. Wants to be on the move._

Speech patterns/content
Talks rather quickly. Repetitious, mispronounces words.

Mood
Appears tense, worried. But tries to put on a brave face.

Orientation _Disorientation a potential problem, if level reaches stage of panic._

Patient's understanding of illness _____
Places emphasis on physical symptoms. Particularly conscious of heart beating.

Patient's family's attitudes to patient's illness _____
Parents are concerned. They thought Rebecca might have something physically wrong.

PRESENT PHYSICAL CONDITION

Result of physical examination
Has been examined by Dr Ludlow. No physical cause for symptoms.

Any physical condition for which the patient is receiving treatment?
None.

Activities for daily living

Nutrition

Appetite *Fair*

Special diet/preferences

Amount of fluid per day

Fluid preferences *Milk shakes*

Elimination

Bowel activity *Regular*

Bladder habit *No problems*

Hygiene

Dentures *No*

Washing Bathing Dressing
No problems

Mobility and safety factors

Vision *Good*

Hearing *Good*

Sleep patterns *Usually wakes up*

Menstrual cycle *Irregular*

Areas of concern to the patient (list numerically)
Present symptoms

Patient's problems identified during interview (list numerically)
Refer to conceptual framework

Further reading

Martin, Ian C. A., Twitch and between. 1. Aspects of the relaxation technique, *Nursing Times*, **74** (23), 953–955, 1978

Martin, Ian C. A., Twitch and between. 2. Further applications of the relaxation technique. *Nursing Times*, **74** (24), 1017–1018, 1978

Martin, Ian C. A., Twitch and between. 3. The relaxation technique in the treatment of illness, *Nursing Times*, **74** (25), 1056–1058, 1978.

Suggested reading

Peplau, H.E., Professional closeness, *Nursing Forum*, **8**(4), 343–360, 1969

Wolf, Z. R., The caring concept and nurse identified caring behaviours, *Topics in Clinical Nursing*, **8** (2), 84–92, 1986

Chapter 2

Nursing the patient who is phobic

Introduction

In phobic anxiety the patient's anxiety is not precipitated by any particular set of circumstances; this is called free-floating anxiety. In phobic anxiety the patient has a fear of a specific object or situation. Spielberger[1] states that phobias tend to endure because they cause a phobic person to avoid the feared object or situation. Thus the patient is prevented from discovering that the object or situation on which his fear is based is really harmless.

Patients will go to extreme and elaborate lengths to avoid the stimulus of their anxiety, e.g. a patient who has a fear of enclosed spaces (claustrophobia) may walk up twelve flights of stairs rather than take the lift.

There are many different types of phobia, e.g. erythrophobia — blushing in public, agoraphobia — fear of open spaces, phonophobia — fear of certain sounds, plus numerous animal and insect phobias.

Serious phobias can have a crippling effect on the individual's life.

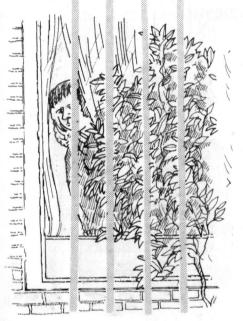

Patient profile

Mrs Ayres, aged 45, was married with a grown-up family. Her confidence diminished when her only daughter left home to get married. She became increasingly anxious whenever she tried to leave the house; eventually her symptoms became so disabling that she was unable to go any further than her own front gate. She became totally dependent on her husband, who had to do all the shopping.

Because Mrs Ayres was unable to go out she became more and more isolated. Friends stopped visiting her as her conversation centred around herself. Her husband lost patience with her and began to lead his own life. Mrs Ayres remained housebound for nearly three years; it was only when her daughter saw a television programme about phobias that she realised that her mother was ill. The GP was consulted and arranged for Mrs Ayres to be seen by a psychiatrist, who referred her to the nurse therapist.

Plan

1. To enable the patient to overcome avoidance behaviour of feared situation.
2. To identify the areas of least and greatest anxiety in order to draw up a desensitisation programme (Figure 2.1).
3. To learn to initiate muscle relaxation.
4. To increase the patient's interaction and social mobility outside the home.

Implementation

The nurse had received some specialised training in behavioural therapy techniques; his first task was to establish rapport with Mrs Ayres and discuss the aims of the treatment programme with her. She was asked to draw up a list of situations which would cause her to be anxious. These were placed in a hierarchy starting with those the patient described as being least anxiety

ASSESSMENT INTERVIEW

(Fill in or delete, as appropriate)

Consultant _Dr Price_

GP _Dr Singh_

Referred by _GP_

Date of referral _15.11.83_ Date of admission _____

Short-stay ward _____

Medium-stay ward _____

Long-stay ward _____

Day hospital _____

Community Nursing Service _X_

Status _____

Surname ~~Mr/Mrs/Miss~~ _Ayres_

Forenames _Veronica_

Address _1 The Close, East Raylton_

Tel. No. _065 3692_

Name of next of kin _Husband Mr Ayres_

Address

As above

Tel. No. _____

Name by which the patient likes to be addressed _Mrs Ayres_

Birthday _14.2.1936_

DESCRIPTION OF THE PATIENT

Colour of eyes _Blue_   Hair colour _Brown/Grey_

Height (m) _1.575_   Weight (kg) _47.6_

Distinguishing features

Small scar left cheek.
Pale complexion.

Present occupation/Occupational history

Housewife
Office work prior to marriage

Hobbies and interests

Homebased. Sewing, Cooking, reading, television

Family or persons of significance in patient's life

Husband, son, married daughter and son in law (Mr and Mrs Shipley)

Persons expected to visit/Support systems

Not relevant

Religion

None

Home conditions

Semi-detached council house. Very clean and tidy. Patient is very house-proud

Community services involved/referred

Name of person _Mr Jan Knapp_

Status _Nurse therapist_

Tel. No. _Ext 521_

Whether contacted (and reason for contacting, if relevant)

Yes. Referred for desensitisation

Psychiatric Condition

Previous psychiatric illness

Handicapped by agoraphobia for nearly three years before any help sought, didn't realise help was available

Present psychiatric condition

General appearance _Neat woman of 'motherly' appearance_

Behaviour _Anxious, unable to relax, expresses her anxiety by the need to be active_

Speech patterns/content _Quietly spoken, talks timidly, mainly about herself_

Mood _Appropriate to situation, only experiences intense anxiety if she has to leave the house_

Orientation _Normal_

Patient's understanding of illness _Feels her problem has got out of hand. Wonders if anything really can be done to help her, after such a long time_

Patient's family's attitudes to patient's illness _Daughter is sympathetic._
Husband is at work when nurse calls and is yet to be seen.

Present Physical Condition

Result of physical examination

General health good, varicose veins both legs, has refused treatment. Primary Raynaud's Syndrome

Any physical condition for which the patient is receiving treatment?

Yes, receiving Tolazoline 25mg three times daily for Primary Raynaud's syndrome

Activities for daily living

Nutrition

Appetite *Good*

Special diet/preferences *None*

Amount of fluid per day *Not known*

Fluid preferences *Tea*

Elimination

Bowel activity *Regular*

Bladder habit *Normal*

Hygiene

Dentures *Yes*

Washing Bathing Dressing
Engages in all these self care activities

Mobility and safety factors

Vision *Reading good with spectacles*

Hearing *Good*

Sleep patterns *Good, usually*

Menstrual cycle *Hysterectomy 6 years ago*

Areas of concern to the patient (list numerically)

Mrs Ayres is concerned that her husband has lost all patience with her. He doesn't understand how panicky she becomes if she tries to go out.

Patient's problems identified during interview (list numerically)

1. The patient has not left her home for nearly three years.

2. Any attempt to do so results in extreme anxiety.

3. She has become socially isolated.

4. Depends on her husband to do all the household shopping, buys other items from mail order.

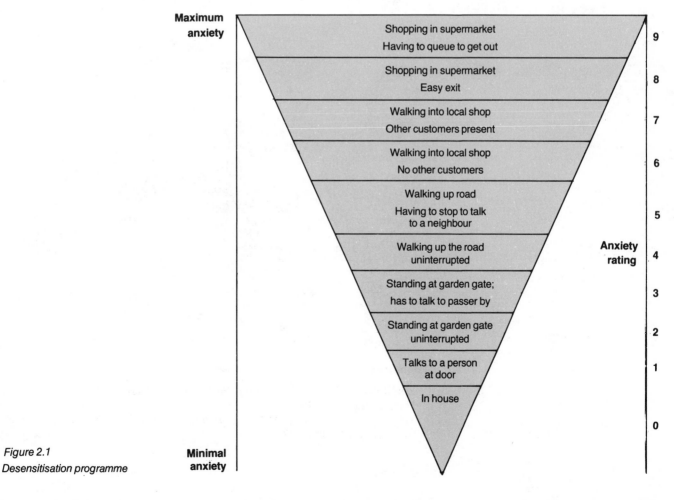

Figure 2.1
Desensitisation programme

29

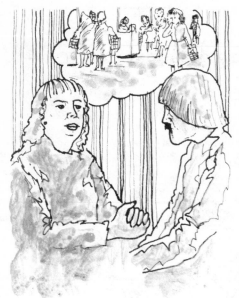

provoking to those which would cause the greatest anxiety. Mrs Ayres was then taught to induce the deep muscle relaxation which she would need to practise at each stage of the therapy. Instead of actually experiencing the real stimulus situation, she was asked to imagine the first situation in the hierarchy after achieving full relaxation. The nurse then moved through the hierarchy of situations with the patient until the situation was reached that brought about the greatest fear response. As Mrs Ayres was still deeply relaxed while imagining her greatest fear, theoretically she was free of her phobia. After this she was able to place herself in the real situation without feeling anxious. Whaley and Malott[2] state that this technique along with other behavioural techniques has made phobic responses a relatively simple problem for the therapist to deal with. Unfortunately the problems of some phobic patients are more complex; this proved to be the case with Mrs Ayres. Her new-found mobility made her a regular attender at her doctor's surgery.

Rationale

Relaxation is incompatible with anxiety.

Evaluation

Mrs Ayres achieved her goals quickly; she overcame her fears of leaving the house; renewed her independence and in turn her opportunities for social interaction.

However, shortly after completing the therapy she complained of feelings of depression and is now being treated by her GP.

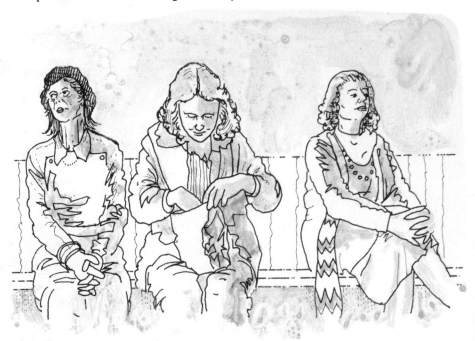

References

1. Spielberger, C., *Understanding Stress and Anxiety, A Life Cycle Series*, Harper and Row, 1979
2. Whaley, D. and Malott, R.W., *Elementary Principles of Behaviour*, Appleton Century Crofts, 1971

Fact sheet: Some common phobias

An exaggerated and pathological fear of:

Animals	Zoophobia	Loneliness	Eremophobia
Bees	Melissophobia	Mirrors	Eisoptrophobia
Blood	Haematophobia	Night	Nyctophobia
Choking	Prigophobia	Odours	Olfactophobia
Disease	Nosophobia	Pain	Algophobia
Dirt	Mysophobia	Reptiles	Ophidiophobia
Eating	Sitophobia	Spiders	Arachnephobia
Fire	Pyrophobia	Thunderstorms	Astraphobia
God	Theophobia	Uncleanliness	Automysophobia
Heights	Acrophobia	Vomiting	Emetophobia
Insanity	Lysophobia	Water	Hydrophobia

Further reading

Campbell, R.J., *Psychiatric Dictionary*, Oxford University Press, 1981
Glossary of Terms and Tests Used in Psychiatric Practice, Lancaster Moor Hospital, 1973

Chapter 3

Nursing the patient who is obsessional

Introduction

Most people have some obsessional traits; they may have a need to straighten hanging pictures, a liking for tidiness and order, or put their milk bottles out in pairs rather than singly. The play activities of children often feature elements of obsessive compulsive behaviour, e.g. touching every lamp post in the street, avoiding cracks in the paving. Adults may show evidence of similar behaviour, e.g. touching wood as a symbol of good luck, or not walking under ladders. The obsessional person is dominated by a need for conformity, order and self-discipline, he is reliable, conscientious and punctual when keeping appointments.

He may adopt fairly rigid routines for daily living, and experience considerable anxiety if these are disrupted by unforeseen circumstances. Having obsessional traits is not a prerequisite for the development of an obsessional compulsive disorder but sometimes this may be the case. When a person develops an obsessive compulsive neurosis the following symptoms may be present:

> Obsessional thoughts and impulses . . ., Recurring thoughts fill the patient's mind and are usually out of keeping with his self-image. The devout churchgoer may have an urge to shout obscene words; the moralistic to shout about a promiscuous sex life. The individual may be in a constant state of doubt. He has to check that he has closed the windows or unplugged the television; he has to check many times often with much inconvenience to himself and others. Even when he has checked that all is well he still remains in doubt.
>
> Some patients have a fear of harming others and may lock up knives and other sharp implements or they may fear they have run someone down when driving, and only drive if they have a passenger who can check for them.

(a) Compulsions

The patient is compelled to carry out a series of actions which provide temporary relief from anxiety, but such is the nature of his illness that having performed his ritualistic acts he is forced to repeat the behaviour over again.

Motor acts may include hand washing, touching some objects and avoiding others, the frequent changing of underwear, wearing gloves to avoid contamination by germs and other complex forms of ritual making. The ritualistic behaviour serves to release the patient's anxiety; he knows it is irrational but an inner compulsion urges him into carrying out these acts. Eventually the illness becomes a terrible handicap; normal life is severely disrupted for the patient and his family.

Occasionally the condition improves spontaneously, but more often patients become depressed and suicidal.

Patient profile

Stephen Hillier was a placid young man in his early 20s. He had recently married and worked as a clerk at the local town hall. After only a few months of marriage Stephen began to change from an easy-going person and started to criticise his wife Julie about the untidiness of their home. Needless to say this brought about a certain amount of friction. Julie had a very casual approach to domestic chores, and tended to give the place a good clean once a week as she had a full-time job.

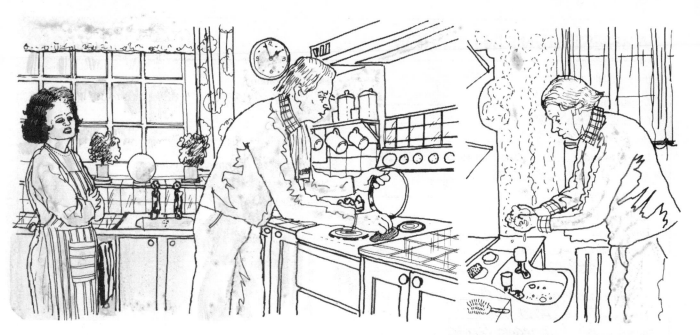

When Stephen came home from work he began to clean and tidy the house. Then the handwashing began; after carrying out small tasks he washed his hands three times. so that everything he did took longer and longer. He began to take a clean shirt and a set of underwear to work which he changed into at lunchtime, he changed them again when he returned home. He was constantly checking windows and appliances, and he always had to go back to make sure the front door was locked when they left for work, despite the fact that Julie assured him that the door was locked.

Julie was finding Stephen's behaviour infuriating; she couldn't even have a good row with him because he never retaliated when she showed anger towards him. She was upset and began to regret her marriage; it wasn't what she was expecting.

Eventually she could take no more and decide to go back to her mother. It was her mother who suggested that perhaps Stephen was ill. The GP was approached and Stephen was persuaded to see a psychiatrist.

Plan

1. Assist Stephen to reduce his anxiety and gain control over actions.
2. Help him to express his feelings.
3. Communicate with, and support, the patient's family.

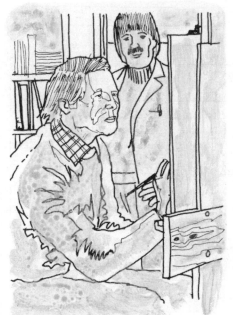

Implementation

Stephen was referred to the nurse therapist for apotrepic therapy. Meyer[1] considered that if a patient could be persuaded to remain in feared situations and could be prevented from carrying out his avoidance rituals, his anxiety would diminish when he learned that the feared consequences do not take place.

Stephen was prevented from engaging in his ritualistic behaviour by persuasion, and diversion when necessary. The prevention of ritualistic behaviour initially resulted in Stephen experiencing high levels of anxiety; the nurse ensured that the time Stephen had previously filled with his ritualistic behaviour was occupied by creative activities.

The nurse recognised Stephen's anxiety and encouraged him to talk about his feelings. She also acted as a model to show him that the expression of anger through socially acceptable channels is a normal healthy response.

ASSESSMENT INTERVIEW

(Fill in or delete, as appropriate)

Consultant _Dr Lyle_
GP _Dr Singh_
Referred by _GP_
Date of referral _____ Date of admission _19.10.83_
Short-stay ward _Reynolds_
Medium-stay ward _____
Long-stay ward _____
Day hospital _____
Community Nursing Service _____
Status _Informal_

Surname Mr/~~Mrs~~/~~Miss~~ _Hillier_
Forenames _Stephen John_
Address _66 Kitchener Terrace,_
East Raylton

Tel. No. _No_
Name of next of kin _Wife Julie_
Address _As above_

Tel. No. _____
Name by which the patient likes to be addressed _Stephen_
Birthday _24.5.1958_

DESCRIPTION OF THE PATIENT

Colour of eyes _Grey blue_ Hair colour _Light Brown_
Height (m) _1.676_ Weight (kg) _63.5_

Distinguishing features
Fair complexion, clean shaven, prominent nose

Present occupation/Occupational history
Clerk, since leaving school. Borough of Raylton

Hobbies and interests
Spends time at local museums, calligraphy and reads

Family or persons of significance in patient's life
Parents, wife, and mother-in-law, also elder brother

Persons expected to visit/Support systems
All above

Religion
Methodist

Home conditions
Small modernised terraced house

Community services involved/referred
Name of person _Mr Jan Knapp_
Status _Nurse therapist_
Tel. No. _Ext 521_
Whether contacted (and reason for contacting, if relevant)
Yes

Psychiatric Condition

Previous psychiatric illness
Received anti-depressant drugs from GP six years ago for mild depression

Present psychiatric condition
General appearance _Appears tense and apprehensive. Neatly dressed_

Behaviour _Obsessive compulsive behaviour, washing rituals, needs to change shirt and underwear 3 times a day_

Speech patterns/content _Accelerated speech_

Mood _Anxious_

Orientation _Normal_

Patient's understanding of illness _Knows his behaviour is irrational, but feels compelled to carry out his rituals_

Patient's family's attitudes to patient's illness _Wife is supportive to husband now that she knows he is suffering from an illness, and has returned to the marital home_

Present Physical Condition

Result of physical examination

Health good, but some recent weight loss

Any physical condition for which the patient is receiving treatment?

None

Activities for daily living

Nutrition

Appetite _Fairly good_

Special diet/preferences _Vegetarian (so is wife)_

Amount of fluid per day _1–2 litres_

Fluid preferences _Apple juice_

Elimination

Bowel activity _Regular_

Bladder habit _Normal_

Hygiene

Dentures _No_

Washing Bathing Dressing
Excessive hand washing

Mobility and safety factors

Vision _Good_

Hearing _Good_

Sleep patterns _Disturbed pattern_

Menstrual cycle _N/A_

Areas of concern to the patient (list numerically)

Worried about the effects of his illness on his wife and their relationship

Patient's problems identified during interview (list numerically)

1. A need to clean and tidy the house each evening.
2. Washes hands three times after any minor task.
3. Constantly checks doors, windows and appliances.
4. Changes underwear, shirt and socks three times a day.
5. Marital disharmony related to present behaviour.
6. Patient is unable to express anger.

Rationale

The nurse helps the patient to regain control over his actions.

Evaluation

Stephen was encouraged to abstain from engaging in ritualistic behaviour. Initially he required continuous supervision by nursing staff; this supervision was gradually withdrawn as he improved. However, at one period Stephen became uncooperative and resumed his washing rituals. Supervision was increased until this behaviour diminished.

Stephen's relationship with Julie has improved, especially as she now understands that his behaviour was the result of an illness. He feels more able to discuss his innermost feelings with her instead of bottling them up.

Stephen has now been discharged and has returned to work. He has been seen as an out-patient once, and was pleased to report that there has been no further ritualistic behaviour. He has complained about sexual problems between himself and Julie. The Consultant has made an appointment to see them jointly with a view to referring the couple to a Marriage Guidance Counsellor.

Reference

1. Meyer, V., Modification of expectations in cases with obsessional rituals, *Behaviour, Research and Therapy*, **4**, 373–380. In: Beech, H.R. and Vaughan, M. (Eds), *Behavioural Treatment of Obsessional States*, Wiley, 1966.

Chapter 4

Nursing the patient who is attention-seeking

Introduction

The nursing student will probably have met in her daily life individuals who like to be the focus of attention. They may be self-centred, manipulative and prone to sulking when they are unable to get their own way. They may lack any loyalty or sensitivity towards the needs of others, and hide their shallow feelings by displays of spurious emotion. When such personality traits are exaggerated the person may be described as suffering from a hysterical personality; such a personality is not necessarily a prerequisite for a psychiatric illness, but the nurse will most certainly meet patients who exhibit attention-seeking behaviour; they are usually in hospital for a variety of other reasons.

The hysterical personality is aptly described by Jaspers[1] who wrote that the hysterical personality seems to have lost its core and to consist entirely of a series of shifting masks.

The nursing student may also meet patients suffering from hysterical neurosis of which there are two main types:

1. Conversion hysteria.
2. Dissociative reactions.

(a) Conversion hysteria

In conversion hysteria an emotional conflict is unconsciously represented by a physical symptom. Such a disability can be manifest in many different ways, e.g. deafness, blindness, convulsions, loss of voice or hoarseness, visceral dysfunctions and paralysis.

The condition of conversion hysteria has been called the great imitator, because of the many forms of disability which may be presented. The patient's symptoms always follow his idea of how his body works and not the rules of anatomy and physiology. Despite the severity of the disability the patient acts with complacency or unconcern. This is called 'La Belle Indifference'.

(b) Dissociative reactions

These are departures from the normal state of consciousness. The individual splits off part of his conscious awareness in an attempt to deal with his anxiety. Dissociative phenomena can be expressed in four ways:

1 Amnesia

Loss of memory which can last for hours, days or even years. The individual cannot remember his name, where he lives or anything about his previous life. Intellectual or manual skills are not usually lost.

2 Fugue states

The patient removes himself from a stressful situation to another place but has no recollection of the journey.

3 Somnambulism

Sleep-walking — when the individual is asleep the split portion of his personality takes over.

4 Multiple personality

The presence of quite separate and different personalities within one individual.

Patient profile

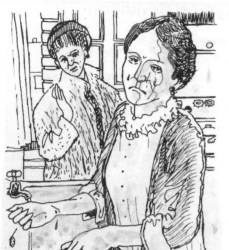

Greta was born in 1954, an illegitimate child. Her early years were spent with various foster parents. Her mother married when she was nearly four and she went to live with her. The marriage however was short-lived: there were frequent quarrels and Greta's stepfather left home. Her mother then started to drink heavily and Greta was eventually taken into care again. When she was eight she was adopted by a large jovial lady, whom she called Aunt Wilma.

Aunt Wilma thoroughly spoilt and cossetted Greta; she loved to dress her up in pretty new clothes. Throughout her childhood Greta never really made any friends of long standing. Her friendships were very superficial. She left school and worked for a while on a factory assembly line. When she was eighteen she met Ron at work, whom she later married.

Ron was a kind person of a rather meek disposition, he soon learned that Greta could make life very difficult if she didn't get her own way. Greta liked to go out dancing in the evenings; she always wanted something new to wear. Greta didn't want any children, Ron did, but even more he wanted to please her. Greta was very attractive and Ron always considered he was very lucky to have married her. On Greta's 21st birthday Aunt Wilma died suddenly; Greta retired to her bed for a week; she didn't attend the funeral. Shortly after this she consulted her doctor because she felt depressed. Since then she has had six admissions to the psychiatric unit. She was last discharged six months ago and has had the regular support of the Community Psychiatric Nurse, Mrs Bryant.

Greta demanded a great deal of the nurse's time; recently she had used vague suicidal threats to arouse her concern. One morning Greta rang Mrs Bryant demanding an immediate visit. The nurse was unable to call at once, but promised to call later in the day. When she arrived she found Greta in a tearful state; she had made several superficial cuts to her wrist. The nurse contacted the appropriate bodies and arranged for Greta's admission.

A diagnosis of depression in a hysterical personality was made.

ASSESSMENT INTERVIEW

(Fill in or delete, as appropriate)

Consultant _Dr Foster_

GP _Dr Kaufert_

Referred by _GP_

Date of referral _____ Date of admission _13.4.83_

Short-stay ward _Landseer_

Medium-stay ward _____

Long-stay ward _____

Day hospital _____

Community Nursing Service _✓_

Status _Informal_

Surname ~~Mr/Mrs/Miss~~ _Green_

Forenames _Greta Emma_

Address _14 Church Street, Raylton_

Tel. No. _060 0214_

Name of next of kin _Husband Mr Ron Green_

Address _As above_

Tel. No. _____

Name by which the patient likes to be addressed _Greta_

Birthday _14.6.1954_

DESCRIPTION OF THE PATIENT

Colour of eyes _Brown_   Hair colour _Auburn_

Height (m) _1.63_   Weight (kg) _44.5_

Distinguishing features

Petite woman, youthful appearance, tanned skin

Present occupation/Occupational history

Factory worker
Cashier in supermarket
Now housewife

Hobbies and interests

Dancing, cinema, television, reads women's magazines. Spends considerable time keeping her tan in summer in her garden, other times uses sun bed which husband bought

Family or persons of significance in patient's life

Husband
Mrs Carole Cater, close friend

Persons expected to visit/Support systems

The above

Religion

None

Home conditions

Pleasant ground floor flat in Edwardian villa. House divided up some years ago by council who took over the property. Husband works 5 minutes walk away, he is able to go home for lunch every day

Community services involved/referred

Name of person _Mrs Bryant_
Status _Community Psychiatric Nurse_
Tel. No. _Ext 3330_

Whether contacted (and reason for contacting, if relevant)
Arranged patient's admission

Psychiatric Condition

Previous psychiatric illness

Six previous admissions to psychiatric unit, on last three times following a small overdose of drugs

Present psychiatric condition

General appearance _Smartly dressed, pays great attention to detail, wears a lot of eye make up_

Behaviour _Draws attention to herself, childish and immature_

Speech patterns/content _Giggly, uses little-girl voice_

Mood _Mildly depressed, sulky when she cannot obtain her own way, sometimes tearful_

Orientation _Normal_

Patient's understanding of illness _Says she is fed up - that's all._
Life has been very unfair to her

Patient's family's attitudes to patient's illness _Husband is very tolerant of patient's demanding behaviour_

Present Physical Condition

Result of physical examination
General health good

Any physical condition for which the patient is receiving treatment?
None

Activities for daily living

Nutrition

Appetite _Fair_

Special diet/preferences _Doesn't eat eggs_

Amount of fluid per day _1½ litres_
Fluid preferences _Coffee only_

Elimination

Bowel activity _Normal_
Bladder habit _Normal_

Hygiene

Dentures _No_

Washing   Bathing   Dressing
No assistance needed - bathes frequently

Mobility and safety factors

Vision _Good_
Hearing _Normal_
Sleep patterns _Never goes to bed until after midnight. Normally late riser_

Menstrual cycle _Pre-menstrual tension_
Always gets headaches prior to a period

Areas of concern to the patient (list numerically)

'You will stop me from doing something silly won't you nurse? Ron doesn't love me any more, that's why I did it. I want to end it all'

Patient's problems identified during interview (list numerically)

1. Attention seeking behaviour shown by:
   (a) Refusal of food
   (b) Inability to swallow hard food
   (c) Request for special soft diet
   (d) Vague threat of suicide
2. May be rejected by some members of staff who find her behaviour difficult to accept.
3. Has tendency to manipulate others in order to get her own way.
4. Displays dependency.

Plan

1. To encourage mature independent behaviour.
2. To promote positive staff attitudes towards Greta.

3. To guard against manipulation.
4. To provide the elements of care necessary for the patient's depressed mood.
5. To fulfil Greta's need for attention through purposeful activity and responsibility.

Implementation

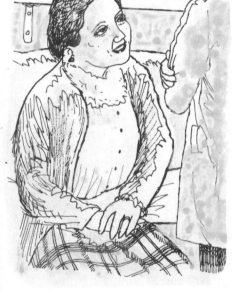

Greta expressed her attention-seeking behaviour by the refusal of food when she was unable to receive something 'special' from the hospital kitchen. She even persuaded some of the other patients to purchase items of food for her from the hospital shop. The nurse attempted to reduce the opportunities for Greta's manipulative behaviour; she was aware that such behaviour is more likely to occur when the patient feels she is behaving well, yet receiving no praise for her good behaviour. Therefore when Greta engaged in mature behaviour this was reinforced by rewarding responses; whereas undesirable behaviour was not reinforced at all. When the nurse found Greta's behaviour annoying, she attempted to understand not only the underlying reasons for the behaviour but also the reaons for her own negative feelings. Lancaster[2] writes that nurses need to be aware of their own emotions if the relationship is to be therapeutic.

Greta's need for attention was met by giving her a small area of responsibility; she was asked to help an elderly patient to the dining room at mealtimes. Unfortunately she soon tired of this, so the nurse decided to deploy Greta's talents in organising the patients' social. Greta was quite successful at this, as it provided her with a sense of importance and usefulness.

Greta liked men, especially male nurses to whom she behaved seductively. The male nurses were always careful to make non-sexual responses towards her and interact with Greta within the group context. Greta particularly benefited from psychodrama, which is a method of psychotherapy. She was encouraged to express her feelings freely through the medium of acting, in the hope that this would assist her to gain insight into her problem by developing a more realistic view of herself. The nurse encouraged Greta to discuss her feelings following these sessions and promoted more mature behaviour through self-discovery. Greta's depressed mood lifted. It was noted that she didn't make suicidal threats when she was engaged in carrying out and enjoying her allocated responsibilities. Nevertheless her threats were not taken lightly, and she was observed all the time.

Perhaps the most useful change in Greta's lifestyle would be for her to obtain a job so that she would be engaged in some purposeful activity. This suggestion was put to Greta, but she was not very enthusiastic initially about the idea.

The Community Psychiatric Nurse will encourage Greta to develop interests outside the home when she is discharged.

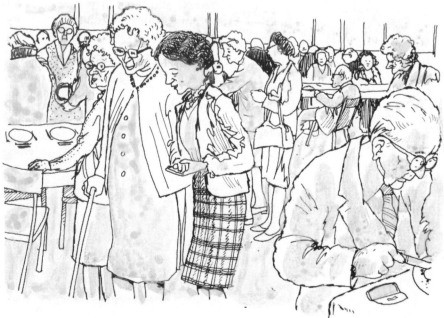

Rationale

The nurse accepts the patient as she is and attempts to modify her behaviour through an understanding of her underlying problems.

Evaluation

The nurses guarded against Greta's manipulation by careful communication both with the patient and among themselves when giving and receiving reports.

Some nurses found difficulty in relating to Greta because of their own negative attitudes towards her. More positive approaches were encouraged through open discussions at ward meetings and by adhering to nursing goals.

Greta's behaviour became less egocentric and she became more thoughtful and considerate towards others. Even her husband commented on this after she had been home for weekend leave.

The Community Psychiatric Nurse who had been involved with Greta prior to her admission maintained contact with her during her hospitalisation and will continue to support her now that she has been discharged. She will encourage Greta to reach the outstanding goals.

References

1. Jaspers, K., in Sainsbury, M.J., *Key to Psychiatry*, H. M. and M. Publishers, 3rd edn, 1980
2. Lancaster, J., *Adult Psychiatric Nursing*, Medical Examination Publishing Co, 1980

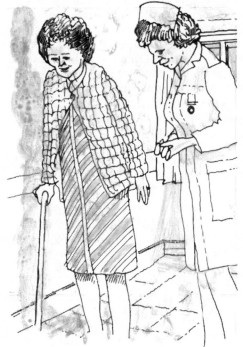

Patient profile

Mrs Manningwood Smith, aged 48, lived in a pleasant middle class suburb. Her husband was a solicitor and they had three children. The eldest son was married and worked in his father's practice. Her second son, a journalist, lived and worked abroad. The youngest child, a daughter, was completing her final year at university.

Mrs Manningwood Smith felt closer to Marlene than either of her sons or her husband; she looked forward to the vacations when Marlene was at home. It was rather a shock when Marlene rang to say she had met someone at university and was going to marry him. The family had always assumed that Marlene would marry a local surgeon's son. The two families had been friendly for a number of years. Marlene brought her husband-to-be home to meet her parents and Mrs Manningwood Smith took an instant dislike to him, finding him gregarious and outspoken, worse still he came from a totally different background. He was definitely not the kind of husband she had in mind for her daughter!

Several weeks after the meeting Mrs Manningwood Smith lost the use of the left side of her body, although there was no facial paralysis. She was admitted to the local hospital; after extensive tests there was no evidence of any cerebral lesion. A psychiatric opinion suggested a diagnosis of conversion hysteria. The Consultant saw the patient's husband and suggested that his wife could benefit from psychiatric care. Mr Manningwood Smith demanded a second opinion and it was only after this that he reluctantly agreed to his wife's transfer.

Plan

1. To seek to discover the patient's underlying problem and to assist her to reach a satisfactory solution.
2. To avoid increasing secondary gain factors.
3. To promote positive attitudes among staff.
4. To provide avenues of support for the patient's family.

ASSESSMENT INTERVIEW

(Fill in or delete, as appropriate)

Consultant _Dr Sands_
GP _Dr Longford_
Referred by _Dr Khedun_
Date of referral _____ Date of admission _12.11.83_
Short-stay ward _Constable_
Medium-stay ward _____
Long-stay ward _____
Day hospital _____
Community Nursing Service _____
Status _Informal_

Surname Mr/Mrs/Miss _Manningwood Smith_
Forenames _Moira Emma_
Address _The Vines, Haynes Lane, Raylton_

Tel. No. _01 060 3911_
Name of next of kin _Mr Sydney Manningwood Smith_
(Husband)
Address _As above_
Tel. No. _____
Name by which the patient likes to be addressed _Moira_
Birthday _17.7.35_

DESCRIPTION OF THE PATIENT

Colour of eyes _Green_   Hair colour _Black_
Height (m) _1.676_   Weight (kg) _63.5_

Distinguishing features
Well groomed, hair highlighted with blue streaks

Present occupation/Occupational history
Housewife, member of various voluntary societies

Hobbies and interests
Reading, embroidery, gardening

Family or persons of significance in patient's life
Children and husband

Persons expected to visit/Support systems
Family, family friends, Rev Parker, St.Lukes

Religion
Church of England, active churchgoer

Home conditions
Large detached house in the best area of Raylton. Does her own cooking, has assistance in the garden and employs a part time domestic

Community services involved/referred
Name of person _NIL_
Status _____
Tel. No. _____
Whether contacted (and reason for contacting, if relevant)
_____

Psychiatric Condition

Previous psychiatric illness
No previous psychiatric history

Present psychiatric condition
General appearance _Smartly dressed well nourished patient who looks younger than her 48 years_

Behaviour _Walks slowly leaning heavily on sticks, arouses sympathy among other patients_

Speech patterns/content _A pleasant articulate woman_

Mood _Expresses a mood of unconcern about her condition_

Orientation _Normal_

Patient's understanding of illness _Seen in physical terms_

Patient's family's attitudes to patient's illness _Concerned but critical of nursing staff, may find it difficult to tolerate 'psychiatric label' rather than 'physical label', i.e. stroke_

Present Physical Condition

Result of physical examination

No organic cause found for her condition

Any physical condition for which the patient is receiving treatment?

Takes prescribed analgesics for occasional migraine

Activities for daily living

Nutrition

Appetite _Good_

Special diet/preferences _Has to watch weight/ likes plenty of salads_

Amount of fluid per day _1 litre_

Fluid preferences _Low calorie drinks_

Elimination

Bowel activity _Regular_

Bladder habit _Normal_

Hygiene

Dentures _None_

Washing Bathing Dressing
Expects assistance because of her stroke

Mobility and safety factors

Vision _Good_

Hearing _Good_

Sleep patterns _Usually late retiring_

Menstrual cycle _N/A_

Areas of concern to the patient (list numerically)

Indifferent to her condition, told the nurse 'Oh well I'll have to learn to live with it, won't I ?'

Patient's problems identified during interview (list numerically)

1. Primary gain factor - a physical symptom, i.e. left hemiplegia for which no organic cause can be found. The symptom is representative of an unconscious conflict.

2. Secondary gain factor - legitimised sick role. Attention and concern of family.

3. Critical attitudes of family towards nursing staff.

Implementation

It was essential for the nurse caring for Mrs Manningwood Smith to understand that her behaviour was unconsciously motivated and that her symptom provided her with temporary relief from her problems. The symptom of paralysis also provided the patient with certain advantages, which are termed the secondary gain factors. Primarily, the symptom relieved the patient from a difficult situation and, secondly, her family were very concerned about her.

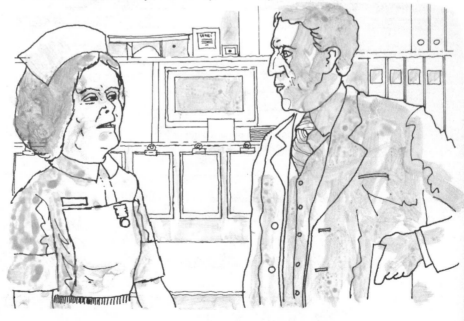

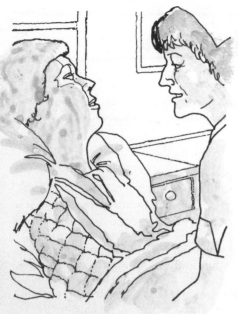

Mrs Manningwood Smith did not deliberately plan her illness. Had she been aware of the beneficial affects of her illness this would have been called malingering, and this is not the same as conversion hysteria.

It requires a nurse with a very positive approach to care for a patient with conversion hysteria. It is probably better if such labels are avoided altogether. Among some nurses the word hysteria can arouse feelings of disapproval, hostility and a feeling that the patient's behaviour is false. Such an attitude can block any attempt to understand the patient's underlying problems.

The nurse did not pay any undue attention to the patient's symptoms, as it was essential not to reinforce them, however, she observed the symptoms closely in order to monitor the patient's progress.

Lancaster[1] writes that a good rule of thumb is to ignore the symptom but never the patient.

Instead of trying to get the paralysed patient to walk, the nurse should try to discover the psychological need for the paralysis. Having established a relationship with Mrs Manningwood Smith the nurse spent time listening to what she had to say. She was encouraged to carry out her own self-care programme and participate in ward activities.

The diagnosis of a psychiatric illness proved to be devastating to the patient's family, particularly her husband. He projected much of his own anxiety and anger on the nursing staff in the form of complaints about his wife's care. Mainly he felt the nursing staff should be doing more for her; he was unable to accept the explanations that this would be contrary to the objectives set for her. The nurse understood the underlying reasons for Mr Manningwood Smith's behaviour, and by remaining objective and supportive attempted to help him to come to terms with his wife's illness.

Rationale

By caring for the patient and *not* her symptoms, the nurse assists her to come to terms with her underlying problems.

Evaluation

The nurses tried to focus their interest on the patient. However, not all the nurses were able to achieve this objective immediately because of their own negative feelings towards the patient. They were encouraged to discuss these feelings openly in a milieu of understanding in order to promote a more positive approach to the patient.

Mrs Manningwood Smith was encouraged to discuss her problems with the nurses; most of the time she denied any psychological problems and viewed her 'paralysis' as something she would have to learn to live with. The staff endeavoured to understand Mr Manningwood Smith's attitude towards his wife's condition. Obviously he found it difficult to accept his wife's illness in psychiatric terms and was instrumental in discontinuing her treatment.

Whenever goals are planned for patients their achievement can be difficult without the support and cooperation of the patient's family, whose behaviours are often based on their own unconscious hopes and fears.

Reference

1. Lancaster, J., *Adult Psychiatric Nursing,* Medical Examination Publishing Co, 1980

Chapter 5

Nursing the patient who is depressed

Introduction

Most people experience feelings of sadness at some time during their lives. It is usually related to some kind of loss or disappointment, and as such is not an abnormal state.

Depression only becomes an illness when the mood is inappropriate in its intensity and duration and interferes significantly with the person's daily life. Depression is one of the commonest psychiatric disorders, the incidence being higher among women. Like anxiety, depression affects the systems of the body and complaints of somatic disturbance are common. These include headache, fatigue, loss of appetite, constipation and sleep disturbances. A diurnal variation accounts for the patient feeling worse at some time during the day. The condition is not always easy to recognise, either by the patient himself or by those he approaches for help; quite a large number of individuals are treated for the physical symptoms which mask their depression. The two main types of depression are:

Reactive Depression
Endogenous Depression

Reactive depression is thought to be related to some significant loss in the person's life, either past or present. The onset of the illness is influenced by environmental factors.

The majority of patients with reactive depression are treated in the community by their GPs, additional support being provided when necessary by the community psychiatric nursing service or attendance at a day hospital.

The symptoms in endogenous depression are usually of such severity that the patient requires a period of hospitalisation. The term endogenous depression denotes a condition which arises from within, environmental influences playing a less important role. There is a distortion of reality, delusions and more rarely hallucinations may be present.

Involutional melancholia is a term used to describe a depressive illness occurring between the ages of 45 and 65 years. It is accompanied by agitation and in women may be associated with the menopause.

The main difference between reactive and endogenous depression is one of degree.

Patient profile

Carole Blunt, age 25, recently moved with her husband from the East End of London to a new town. They had lived in a small upstairs flat ever since they married but it was difficult negotiating the narrow stairs now that they had two small children.

One day Mike announced that his firm were opening a factory in a new town. If he moved they would be rehoused; it seemed like an ideal opportunity. There were parks and open spaces for the children to play; modern schools and shops. Carole had been quite excited at the prospect of moving; she had had some regrets of course, she wouldn't see her parents or Mike's mother as often, and she would miss the friendly atmosphere of the East End.

Carole loved the new house; it was light and spacious. She considered herself very lucky and felt she now had everything she could possibly want. But within a week or two she began to feel very lonely. It wasn't the same as the old community, people weren't as friendly. They seemed to shut themselves away behind the shield of white drapes which adorned each window.

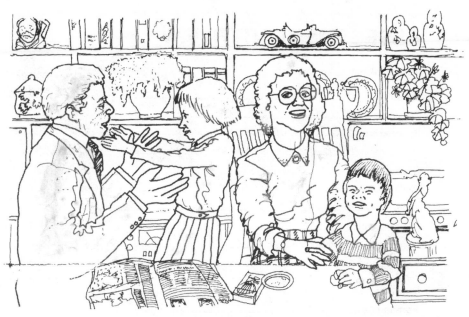

Carole began to develop headaches. She lost interest in sex and her relationship with Mike began to suffer. She couldn't understand what she had to feel miserable about; he didn't help matters by telling her to pull herself together. Sometimes Carole felt very irritable towards the children. When Ian spilt some paint on the new carpet she hit him with such force that he banged his head on the radiator. She was frightened by her own lack of control. She felt she had reached breaking point. She plucked up the courage to go and see her new GP who prescribed some valium for her.

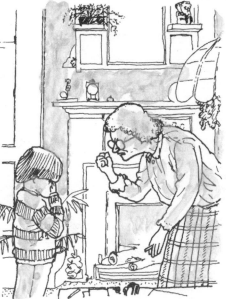

The GP also arranged for a Health Visitor, Mrs Hanson, to pay Carole an early visit. Carole found she could talk to her although she was afraid Mrs Hanson might think she wasn't a very suitable person to be a parent. But the Health Visitor was very aware of the sense of isolation some young mothers experienced in new towns. She discussed Carole's problems with the GP. It was felt that Carole's depression could be managed successfully within the family unit providing she received adequate support. The Community Psychiatric Nurse was asked to visit Carole to provide counselling and support.

Plan

1. To support Carole and her family during the present crisis.
2. To observe her for any signs of increasing depression.
3. To help Carole's husband to appreciate her feelings.
4. To arrange for Ian to attend a play group.
5. To introduce Carole to a young mother's group.

Implementation

When two members of the community health team are engaged in the care of one person good communication is essential. This is best achieved through regular informal meetings. Each member of the health team should have an understanding of the other's role and their particular areas of expertise.

Although there are some similarities in function, this helps to identify the areas of professional responsibility more clearly. All members of the health team observe the code of confidentiality. The Health Visitor is concerned with the prevention of physical and emotional ill health. She detects and practises surveillance of 'at risk' groups, increases her support to families during stressful periods, and mobilises other sources of help when necessary.

ASSESSMENT INTERVIEW

(Fill in or delete, as appropriate)

Consultant _Dr Foster_

GP _Dr Irons_

Referred by _Health visitor_

Date of referral _21·6·83_ Date of admission _____

Short-stay ward _____

Medium-stay ward _____

Long-stay ward _____

Day hospital _____

Community Nursing Service ___X___

Status _____

Surname ~~Mr/Mrs/Miss~~ _Blunt_

Forenames _Carole Jane_

Address _74 Millfield, Raylton New Town_

Tel. No. _No_

Name of next of kin _Husband_

Address _As above_

Tel. No. _No_

Name by which the patient likes to be addressed _Carole_

Birthday _28·4·56_

DESCRIPTION OF THE PATIENT

Colour of eyes _Blue_ Hair colour _Fair_

Height (m) _1·575_ Weight (kg) _51·25_

Distinguishing features
Fair short hair
Looks younger than her 25 yrs. Wears spectacles

Present occupation/Occupational history
Machinist, clothing factory until marriage and birth of first child. Now housewife

Hobbies and interests
Television, making her children's and her own clothes

Family or persons of significance in patient's life
Husband Mike, aged 28, children Ian, aged 4 and Wendy, aged 2½

Persons expected to visit/Support systems
Carole's parents Mr and Mrs Swann
Mike's parents Mr and Mrs Blunt
Parents visit alternate weekends

Religion
None

Home conditions
New open-plan three bedroomed house rented from New Town Development Authority. Enclosed garden at rear for children to play in. Moved into the area three months ago from East London

Community services involved/referred

Name of person _Mrs M. Hanson_

Status _Health Visitor_

Tel. No. _006 1515 Ext 36_

Miss V. Pope
Community Psychiatric Nurse
Ext 3330

Whether contacted (and reason for contacting, if relevant)

_____

Psychiatric Condition

Previous psychiatric illness
None

Present psychiatric condition

General appearance _Clean and tidily dressed. Appears to be tense and anxious. Smokes incessantly_

Behaviour _Tearful, dislikes being alone. Finds concentration difficult. Gets irritable with children, and says she has lost all her confidence_

Speech patterns/content _Keen to talk about her problems_

Mood _Depressed, feels better if in company_

Orientation _Normal_

Patient's understanding of illness _Tends to blame her husband because he is very settled in his new job and can't understand how she feels_

Patient's family's attitudes to patient's illness _Mike can't understand why Carole is depressed now that they have a better lifestyle_

Present Physical Condition

Result of physical examination

_____

_____

Any physical condition for which the patient is receiving treatment?

_____ *None* _____

_____

Activities for daily living

Nutrition

Appetite _____ *Fair*

Special diet/preferences *Dislikes spicey foods*

_____

Amount of fluid per day _____ *2 litres*

Fluid preferences _____ *Plenty of tea*

Elimination

Bowel activity _____ *Normal*

Bladder habit _____ *Normal*

Hygiene

Dentures _____ *No*

Washing Bathing Dressing *Carries out these activities, but neglectful of personal appearance*

Mobility and safety factors

Vision _____ *Wears spectacles*

Hearing _____ *Good*

Sleep patterns *Difficulty in getting to sleep recently*

Menstrual cycle _____ *Regular*

Areas of concern to the patient (list numerically)

1. That she will lose her temper and harm her son.

2. She sees little prospect of feeling better in 'cold unfriendly town.'

3. Wishes her husband understood how she feels.

Patient's problems identified during interview (list numerically)

1. Carole's depression appears to result from a loss of support in a new and strange environment.

2. She is lonely and has a sense of isolation

3. Irritability towards children could be potentially harmful.

4. Her husband seems to lack an understanding of her real problems.

Clark[2] describes her most important and fundamental skills in communication, in establishing and maintaining interpersonal relationships, listening and interpreting, counselling and most importantly, teaching. By arranging for Ian to attend a play group, it will give him the opportunity to mix with other children and to release much of his energy through play activities. It would allow Carole a breathing space in which to adjust to a new way of life.

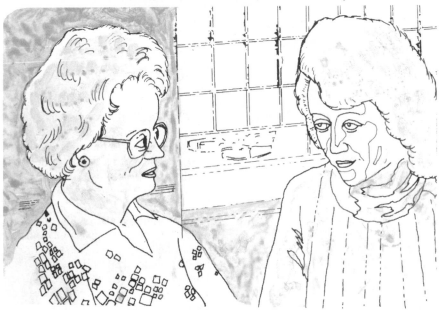

Carole was a newcomer in an alien environment. She felt a sense of isolation and loss in moving from an environment which embraced significant interpersonal relationships and gave her a sense of belonging. Littlefield[1] points out that territorial loss through relocation can have a considerable impact on the displaced person.

The Health Visitor and Community Psychiatric Nurse in their respective roles assisted Carole to adapt to her new environment.

Because there are a number of mothers in new towns who feel similarly isolated the Health Visitor started a self-help group. An introduction to its members enabled Carole to make friends and gain support from others who had experienced similar problems.

The Community Psychiatric Nurse visited Carole to provide additional support throughout her period of readjustment, and to observe her for any evidence of increasing depression. Some discussion with the patient's husband helped him to perceive his wife's problems more empathically.

Rationale

As Carole becomes integrated into the community new support systems should replace the loss of old ties, and she should feel more secure as an individual and in her roles as wife and mother.

Evaluation

The Community Psychiatric Nurse and the Health Visitor in their respective roles provided support for Carole as she adjusted to her new environment, providing her with the opportunity to extend her support systems. As Carole began to feel more secure, her self-esteem increased and she became more confident in her management of the children. She says her husband now understands how she felt, sexual intercourse has resumed and together they are beginning to make new friends.

Should Carole ever feel depressed again she can either approach her Health Visitor or the Community Psychiatric Nurse.

References

1. Littlefield, C. N., in Bower F. (Ed.), *Nursing and the Concepts of Loss*, Wiley, 1980
2. Clark, J., *Role of the Health Visitor in the Health Team in Action*, BBC Publications, 1974

Patient profile

Mr Ford, aged 63, worked as a factory foreman. He had been with the same company for thirty years. He was a conscientious man who was gradually planning for retirement. He and his wife had recently bought a bungalow and were looking forward to moving when everything was finalised. Recently Mr Ford had been drinking quite heavily; normally he had only the occasional pint. He was also troubled by constipation and inwardly he feared he might have cancer.

One Monday morning he stayed in bed. He said he wasn't ill, he just wanted to be left alone. This behaviour was completely out of character; Mr Ford hadn't had a day's sickness for the past five years. He refused to eat any of the food his wife prepared for him. That night Mrs Ford woke up with an uneasy feeling. The place beside her was empty. She found her husband downstairs sitting in the darkness. She made a cup of tea but he wouldn't touch it. Mr Ford seemed so cold and distant. He mumbled something about having committed a terrible sin and there would be a judgement upon him. Mrs Ford had great difficulty in understanding what he was saying. The following morning the GP was called. He diagnosed an Acute Endogenous Depression. The patient was unwilling to go to hospital so the doctor arranged for Mr Ford to be admitted to hospital under Section 4 of the Mental Health Act 1983.

ASSESSMENT INTERVIEW

(Fill in or delete, as appropriate)

Consultant _Dr Sands_

GP _Dr Kaufert_

Referred by _____

Date of referral _____ Date of admission _15.9.83_

Short-stay ward _Constable_

Medium-stay ward _____

Long-stay ward _____

Day hospital _____

Community Nursing Service _____

Status _Section 4 Mental Health (Amendment) Act 1982_

Surname Mr/Mrs/Miss _Ford_

Forenames _Herbert Arthur George_

Address _73 Milestone Point, Raylton_

_____

Tel. No. _01 060 7521_

Name of next of kin _Mrs Patricia Ford (Wife)_

Address _As above_

_____

Tel. No. _____

Name by which the patient likes to be addressed _Mr Ford_

Birthday _12.9.21_

DESCRIPTION OF THE PATIENT

Colour of eyes _Pale Blue_ Hair colour _Dark Grey_

Height (m) _1.676_ Weight (kg) _73_

Distinguishing features

Grey thin receding hair,
Thin pencil line moustache

Present occupation/Occupational history

Section Foreman, Components factory

Hobbies and interests

Treasurer and committee member,
Raylton Ex-Servicemans Club.
Gardening, growing of prize dahlias

Family or persons of significance in patient's life

Wife and married daughter, three grandchildren

Persons expected to visit/Support systems

All the family, possibly committee members of Mr Ford's Club

Religion

None

Home conditions

Semi-detached well-maintained house, moving to recently bought 'retirement' bungalow. No financial problems

Community services involved/referred

Name of person _None_

Status _____

Tel. No. _____

Whether contacted (and reason for contacting, if relevant)

_____

Psychiatric Condition

Previous psychiatric illness

None... Mr Ford's maternal grandmother committed suicide 1926

Present psychiatric condition

General appearance _Looks depressed, shows no response to happenings within the environment_

Behaviour _Sits motionlessly, head bowed, movements lethargic and slow. Avoids the company of other patients_

Speech patterns/content _Voice is flat... Expresses a desire to be left alone_

Mood _Sad and gloomy, self-destructive_

Orientation _Attention span is poor_

Patient's understanding of illness _No insight into illness_

Patient's family's attitudes to patient's illness _Very concerned, will need a great deal of support throughout Mr Ford's illness_

Present Physical Condition

Result of physical examination

General health good

Any physical condition for which the patient is receiving treatment?

None

Activities for daily living

Nutrition

Appetite _Very poor_

Special diet/preferences _Doesn't like fish or salads_

Amount of fluid per day _2 litres_

Fluid preferences _Tea_

Elimination

Bowel activity _Constipated_

Bladder habit _Normal_

Hygiene

Dentures _Full set_

Washing Bathing Dressing
Does need assistance in all these areas

Mobility and safety factors

Vision _Spectacles_

Hearing _Normal_

Sleep patterns _Poor...Troubled by early waking_

Menstrual cycle _N/A_

Areas of concern to the patient (list numerically)

Difficult to ascertain at present

Patient's problems identified during interview (list numerically)

1. Suicide a very real risk.
2. Feelings of guilt and unworthiness.
3. Depressed mood and loss of interest.
4. Sleep disturbance.
5. Constipation.
6. Loss of appetite.
7. Reduced physical activity.
8. Slowed thought processes.
9. Neglect of personal hygiene.

Plan

1. To prevent suicide by providing a safe environment.
2. To help Mr Ford perceive himself as a worthwhile person.
3. To lessen his feelings of sadness.
4. To promote sleep.
5. To establish a regular bowel habit.
6. To enable him to meet his dietary requirements.
7. To allow time for the patient to express himself and engage in physical activity.
8. To assist him to maintain self-care.
9. To provide the elements of nursing care during electroconvulsive therapy.

Implementation

The risk of suicide is increased when depression is accompanied by feelings of guilt and self-depreciation. Mr Ford was identified as a patient who was suicidal to all members of the ward team; each member of the team then became aware of their responsibilities in maintaining vigilance. Staff were alerted to the possible dangers within the ward environment and the ways in which Mr Ford might attempt to end his life (*see* Fact Sheet, p.50).

Provision of a safe environment was of paramount importance. The nurse tried to ensure that items which could be used as weapons of self-destruction were controlled as far as possible.

She had to ensure that Mr Ford took any medication prescribed for him. As he was reluctant to take his tablets, and may have attempted to store them up and take a lethal dose, it was necessary to examine his mouth to see that he had swallowed the dose.

Robinson[1] writes that the nurse feels awkward doing these things to another adult, but she must keep in mind that she is constantly trying to protect the patient's life.

The desire of Mr Ford to end his own life was a feature of his despair, his poor self-image and feelings of unworthiness.

When he expressed his feelings about suicide, the nurse conveyed her understanding of these feelings as part of his illness, but tried to direct his thoughts more positively towards recovery. When a person is depressed he directs his anger inwards towards himself; Mr Ford needed to be provided with things to do to release this inner tension. Competitive activities were not suitable as these would only enhance his sense of failure.

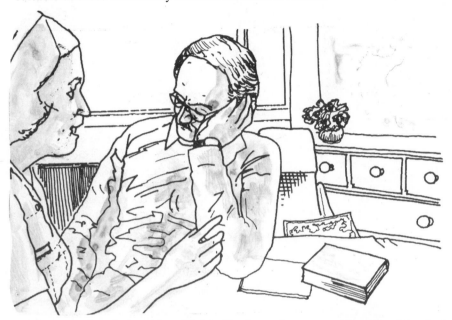

The nurse's relationship with Mr Ford was important in making him feel accepted; she supported him by being with him, and providing quiet companionship. This allowed her the opportunity to observe him closely and to detect any verbal or non-verbal signs about the way he felt. When addressing him she adopted a gentle tone of voice, so as not to increase his awareness of his own sad mood. It was important to listen to what he had to say and to allow him time to express himself, as Mr Ford needed time to gather his thoughts and express them in words.

Sleep is essential to promote physical and mental health; although Mr Ford had no difficulty in getting to sleep he was troubled by early waking. The night nurse manipulated the environment in order to promote sleep; vigilance was never allowed to lapse in the night, because the patient may lie awake contemplating his sense of guilt and unworthiness. Mr Ford's sense of isolation could have led him to attempt suicide; the possibility was always present.

Mr Ford was troubled by constipation and he was given two suppositories to provide immediate relief. The formation of a regular bowel habit was then encouraged by ensuring that he had sufficient fluids, fresh fruit, vegetables and fibre in his diet.

The patient had a poor appetite despite being given small meals; initially he required some assistance with feeding.

He was very reluctant to co-operate in self-care and the nurse had to take over many of these functions on his behalf.

The doctor prescribed a course of electroconvulsive therapy for Mr Ford. He was starved for four hours prior to the treatment in preparation for a general anaesthetic. He was given a careful explanation about the procedure although the word 'electricity' was avoided, because this can sometimes increase a patient's apprehension. The nurse remained with Mr Ford during the treatment and recovery period, ensuring that a clear airway was maintained and that he was positioned correctly.

There was some loss of memory after treatment but this was only temporary. After only two treatments Mr Ford's appetite and general functioning improved considerably.

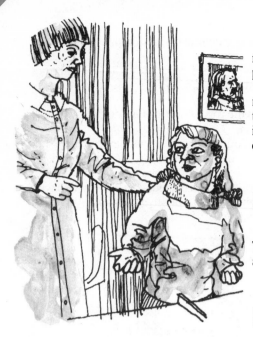

Constant vigilance was still essential; when a patient has been physically retarded and his level of activity improves he may then be in a position to act on previous suicidal intentions.

Mr Ford's wife and daughter needed considerable support; psychiatric illness can make a patient appear like a stranger to his family, and they may feel that they may have contributed in some way. Their own sense of helplessness is increased when the patient refuses to communicate with them, and the nurse can do much to allay their anxiety by bridging this communciation gap.

Rationale

Through her relationship with the patient the nurse can raise his self-esteem and promote recovery.

Evaluation

Mr Ford made a slow recovery initially; after only two electroconvulsive therapy treatments his mental and physical functioning improved considerably. His appetite increased, he was less troubled by early waking and more willing to engage in self-care.

As Mr Ford's depression lifted he became more communicative with the nurses, other patients and more importantly his family who were relieved to see him 'more like his old self'.

The nurses maintained a safe environment for the patient throughout his hospitalisation, and listened closely to what he had to say. He was observed carefully for any indication of suicidal potential, even after he appeared so much better.

Mr and Mrs Ford have now finalised the sale of their own house and will be moving into their bungalow in a matter of weeks.

Mr Ford has now been discharged and will be followed up as an out-patient.

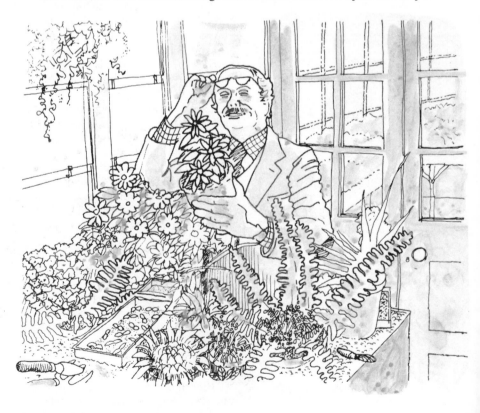

Reference

1. Robinson, L. *Psychiatric Nursing as a Human Experience,* Saunders, 1977

Fact sheet: Nursing the patient who is suicidal

The patient who is suicidal:
1. May not necessarily look sad or miserable.
2. Is often relieved to be able to talk about his feelings, but cannot be considered a lesser risk because he does so.
3. May deny any suicidal thoughts, but this denial cannot be taken as evidence that he does not harbour such ideas.
4. Usually gives others some warning of his intentions through verbal statements and body language.
5. May attempt suicide if he can detect times when the nurse seems to be less watchful, e.g. staff hand-over times, at night when there are fewer staff and at nurse's mealtimes.
6. May present a greater risk if depression is accompanied by guilt feelings, self-depreciation or sleep deprivation.
7. Should be carefully observed when becoming more active after a period of retardation.

Fact sheet: Ways in which a patient may commit suicide

1. Taking an overdose of drugs, e.g. analgesics, antidepressants.
2. Swallowing poison, e.g. bleach, insecticide, acid.
3. Inhaling poisonous fumes, e.g. carbon monoxide.
4. Severing an artery, e.g. throat or wrists.
5. Jumping from a great height.
6. Jumping in front of a moving vehicle.
7. Burning.
8. Electrocution.
9. Suffocation.
10. Shooting.
11. Drowning.
12. Hanging.
13. Starvation.
14. Driving vehicle into stationary object.

Fact sheet: Other conditions which may lead to suicide

1. *The person who is out of touch with reality* may be frightened by his changing thoughts and feelings.
2. *The person who is physically ill* particularly when there is severe or anticipated pain.
3. *The mentally impaired person* may recognise that his mental capacity is deteriorating.
4. *The person who is attention seeking* may wish to gain sympathy or manipulate others.
5. *The drug-dependent person* may seek relief from his problems or wish to spare others from the effects of his addiction.
6. *The psychopathic person* may find his own aggressive impulses difficult to deal with and turn them inward against himself.

Reference

Sharp, D., *Plain Facts — Psychiatric First Aid,* Plain Facts, 1980

Chapter 6

Nursing the patient who is overactive

Introduction

Overactivity may be seen in anxiety, agitation and hyperthyroidism, but the most overactive patient the nurse is likely to encounter is the one suffering from mania or hypomania, the latter being a milder form of the condition.

These patients are mentally and physically overactive. Their conversation changes rapidly from one topic to another. They can be jovial and amusing but this mood can equally be replaced by one of irritability and aggression, especially if they feel that their various plans and schemes are being thwarted by the nursing staff. Normal social constraints are lifted; the patient may make very personal and indiscreet remarks to other patients or staff, little confidences will be conveyed forth for all to hear with embarrassing detail. Sexual desire is increased and this can lead to sexually provocative behaviour.

The patient is full of grandiose ideas which may embrace almost any theme. He is bursting with the energy and enthusiasm to put his ideas into operation. Fortunately one scheme is rapidly dropped for another which takes on equal magnitude and importance. Some patients believe they have enormous wealth, and can bring their family to bankruptcy very quickly with their extravagant spending.

The patient has unbounded confidence in his own ability; however, judgement is completely lacking and the patient must be protected from bringing the harmful consequences of his illness on to himself or his family.

The onset of the illness may pass unrecognised at first by those closest to the patient. His behaviour may be put down to high spirits.

In some patients the elated mood of mania alternates with periods of depression; this is called manic depressive illness. Some patients who have experienced both mood states are able to recognise that they are becoming 'high' but may be reluctant to seek medical assistance. The increasing sense of well-being is enjoyed in contrast to the symptoms of depression.

Fortunately since the advent of psychotherapeutic drugs and electroconvulsive therapy these patients usually respond quite dramatically to treatment.

Patient profile

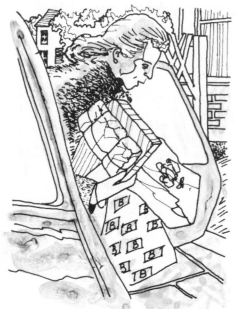

Mary, an only child, spent a happy childhood in the country where her father was a farm bailiff. She was a bright child with a cheerful disposition. She did well at school, gaining good grades in her 'O' level exams. It was Mary's ambition to go to university and eventually become a teacher; her parents however refused Mary help to achieve her ambitions and it was arranged that she should do a secretarial course locally. Mary was very disappointed, but as she enjoyed the course she didn't pursue the idea of university any longer.

When she was eighteen she met John, five years her senior, at a local dance. John had a good job with an insurance company so they married a year later, somewhat against her parent's wishes, and moved to London. Mary continued to work on a part-time basis until their first child was born; within a few days of the birth Mary developed a hypomanic illness. She was in hospital for three months and made a good recovery.

John's mother, a widow, arrived to care for baby James and to support Mary when they left hospital. This Mary was glad of; she enjoyed her mother-in-law's support and company, as she had distanced herself from her own parents since her marriage. Following the birth of her second child, Emma, Mary suffered another similar illness and to assist and give her continued support it was decided that the mother-in-law would sell up her own home and move in with them.

ASSESSMENT INTERVIEW

(Fill in or delete, as appropriate)

Consultant _Dr I Peers_

GP _Dr Hassan_

Referred by _GP_

Date of referral _18.10.83_ Date of admission _18.10.83_

Short-stay ward _Landseer_

Medium-stay ward _____

Long-stay ward _____

Day hospital _____

Community Nursing Service _____

Status _Informal_

Surname ~~Mr~~/Mrs/~~Miss~~ _Smith_

Forenames _Mary Ann_

Address _6 Rutland Close, Raylton, London_

Tel. No. _584 9991_

Name of next of kin _Mr John Smith (Husband)_

Address _As above_

Tel. No. _____

Name by which the patient likes to be addressed _Mary_

Birthday _12.6.45_

DESCRIPTION OF THE PATIENT

Colour of eyes _Green_ Hair colour _Auburn_

Height (m) _1.677_ Weight (kg) _60_

Distinguishing features
Freckles on face and arms

Present occupation/Occupational history
Secretary when first married. Part time office work since youngest child started school in 1971. Recently appointed office supervisor

Hobbies and interests
Cooking, dressmaking, flower arranging and entertaining

Family or persons of significance in patient's life
Husband, Son James age 15, daughter Emma age 12, Mrs Dora Smith, Mother-in-law, Donald and Anne Hayes, Friends

Persons expected to visit/Support systems
All the above

Religion
Church of England. Attends church for special family occasions only

Home conditions
Large detached house, in pleasant residential part of Raylton. Mother-in-law has lived with family

since 1969, assisting with the additional child. More recently looking after the home whilst Mary took on a more responsible job at the office.

Community services involved/referred

Name of person _Mrs George_

Status _Community Psychiatric Nurse_

Tel. No. _Ext 3330_

Whether contacted (and reason for contacting, if relevant)
Yes, to monitor Mary's progress on discharge

Psychiatric Condition

Previous psychiatric illness
Similar illness following the births of both children - was in mother and baby unit. Hypomanic illness diagnosed on both occasions

Present psychiatric condition

General appearance _Has a preference for bright colours which 'clash', make-up is heavily and inexpertly applied_

Behaviour _Extremely active and energetic. A prolific letter writer. Interferes with the activities of other patients and reacts to the slightest stimuli_

Speech patterns/content _Overtalkative; changes topic of conversation so rapidly that it is almost impossible to keep up with the patient's train of thought (flight of ideas)_

Mood _Elated, happy mood, which changes to one of irritability and short temperamental outbursts. Frequently resorts to clang association - using words that rhyme, e.g. Mary Ann had a lamb, ram, sam_

Orientation _Does not recall events that led to admission_

Patient's understanding of illness _Denies being ill. Mary says she has never felt better in her life. Accuses her husband of standing in the way of her ambitions, i.e. setting up a business for the children_

Patient's family's attitudes to patient's illness _Concerned and supportive_

Present Physical Condition

Result of physical examination

General health good

Any physical condition for which the patient is receiving treatment?

None

Activities for daily living

Nutrition

Appetite _Too busy to eat properly_

Special diet/preferences _Needs a high protein, high calorie diet_

Amount of fluid per day _2 litres_

Fluid preferences _Coffee with saccharin_

Elimination

Bowel activity _Carelessly exercised in full view of others_

Bladder habit _Neglects regular emptying_

Hygiene

Dentures _No_

Washing Bathing Dressing _Neglected since onset of illness, removes clothing_

Mobility and safety factors

Vision _Normal_

Hearing _Normal_

Sleep patterns _Disturbed_

Menstrual cycle _Regular – 28-day cycle_

Areas of concern to the patient (list numerically)

None – because of sense of well being 'feels on top of the world'

Patient's problems identified during interview (list numerically)

1. _Elevated mood and increased general activity._
2. _Grandiose ideas._
3. _Embarrasses other patients by tactless and indiscrete remarks._
4. _Disregards personal hygiene._
5. _Neglect of dietary needs._
6. _Bladder and bowel activities carelessly exercised._
7. _Disturbed sleep pattern_

After her recovery she returned to work and remained well until her present illness. Her elevated mood was thought by the family to be related to her recent promotion at the office. However their bank manager, a friend of long standing, drew John's attention to the fact that Mary was writing an unusually large number of cheques for substantial amounts of money. By now John was extremely anxious about his wife's mental health. He approached Dr Hassan, who arranged for Mary to be admitted to hospital.

Plan

1. To provide an environment in which stimulation is reduced to a minimum.
2. To prevent the patient from carrying out grandiose plans by diversional activities.
3. To anticipate the patient's actions and intervene tactfully in situations which could be potentially embarrassing.
4. To ensure the patient takes adequate nutrition and fluids.
5. To encourage attention to personal hygiene.
6. To encourage regular bladder and bowel activity.
7. To promote sleep by manipulation of the environment.
8. To ensure the patient takes prescribed medication.
9. To observe closely and monitor the patient's mood.
10. To prevent aggressive behaviour.
11. To assist the patient to resume her roles within the family.

Implementation

Mary was sedated and nursed in a quiet single room. She was stimulated as little as possible and the nurse did not promote conversation. Crawford and

Buchanan[1] suggest listening to the patient, but making few comments when the patient is excited.

It took some time before the medication had any effect as some patients can tolerate quite high doses of phenothiazines or other drugs. Initially it was difficult to confine Mary to her room. She was very amusing, cracking jokes and puns, but her mood could equally change to one of irritability. The nurse remained calm and consistent in her management of Mary, and never allowed her feelings of exasperation to be conveyed to the patient, through her tone of voice or action. Mary had to be protected because she was ill and others protected from the consequences of her actions.

Caring for the hyperactive patient is both physically and mentally taxing, and requires a high degree of nursing skill. When the patient is being difficult to tolerate, to argue serves no purpose, and may provoke aggressive behaviour. It is always far better to humour the patient. Mary had numerous ideas flowing through her head — many of these were grandiose and of a delusional nature. They related to her feelings of power, superiority and wealth.

Irving[2] describes the patient's grandiose delusions as often being wish fulfilments meant to compensate for his failure or inadequacy.

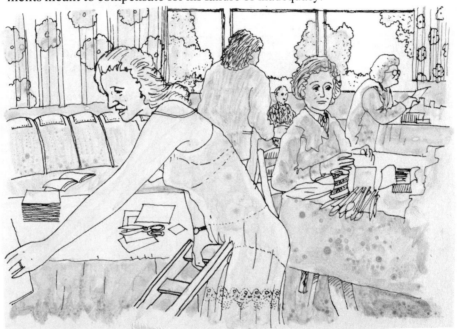

Much of Mary's boundless energy was directed into trying to put her ideas into operational enterprises. One idea was quickly dropped for another, which was pursued with equal tenacity; numerous tasks were started and left unfinished. The nurse tried to divert Mary's attention away from actions which could have harmful consequences; she never forbade Mary from doing something, it was far better to intervene tactfully. Mary had to be encouraged to maintain her personal hygiene at an acceptable level. This was yet another challenge for the nurse as Mary always had more important things to do; when she could be persuaded to have a warm bath this had a relaxing effect.

In caring for Mary's basic needs the nurse had to act as an opportunist. Routines and set meals were not for Mary, the nurse had to choose her moments carefully throughout the day to ensure that Mary had sufficient food and fluids. It was often useful to discover a patient's food preferences but with Mary these changed as rapidly as her other ideas.

Bladder and bowel function presented problems, because Mary was prepared to pass urine or defaecate wherever she stood so the nurse directed her to the toilet at regular intervals.

Mary required night sedation and this was repeated as prescribed. The nurse promoted sleep by reducing environmental stimuli and making the patient as comfortable as possible.

Persuasiveness was essential when giving Mary her medication as she proclaimed that she never felt better in her life and didn't need drugs, but these were necessary to slow her down and prevent the onset of physical exhaustion.

When caring for Mary it was important for the nursing staff to work harmoniously as the patient was highly perceptive in detecting areas of discontent among staff.

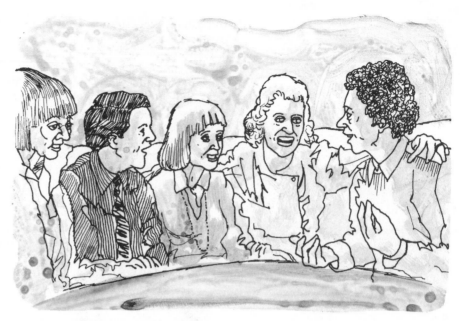

It was explained to Mary's family that she was unable to exert any control over her behaviour, but they were encouraged to support her throughout her illness.

Finally, the nurses were always aware that the patient's elated mood could rapidly change to one of depression.

Rationale

By providing non-stimulating responses the nurse helps to reduce the patient's level of activity.

Evaluation

Mary's changing needs required a frequent review of objectives and the effectiveness of nursing actions in helping her achieve them. It was not found necessary to set new objectives for Mary, but it seemed beneficial for her well-being to concentrate on particular goals at a time to meet the demands of her changing behaviour. At times, for instance, Mary's own safety was paramount; at other times the safety of other patients was more important.

Mary's elevated mood gradually subsided and became within normal limits. She has now been discharged and is due to be seen as an out-patient. She is keen to return to her job as soon as possible, but her husband would like her to stay at home. This is a problem they are trying to resolve between them.

References

1. Crawford, A.L. and Buchanan, B.B., *Psychiatric Nursing — A Basic Manual,* 4th edn, Davis, 1961
2. Irving, S., *Basic Psychiatric Nursing,* Saunders, 1978

Chapter 7 Nursing the patient who is withdrawn

Introduction

Withdrawal can be described as a behaviour pattern in which an individual retreats from relationships or contact with other people. This may be conveyed by adopting a wide range of behaviours. The withdrawn patient may appear aloof, detached and indifferent to his surroundings. He may physically remove himself from the presence of others; adopt a body posture that forbids interaction and avert his gaze when spoken to. He may refuse to engage in spontaneous conversation or only answer with monosyllables; sometimes he may remain mute.

Withdrawal is usually observed in the patient who is out of touch with reality. The patient may feel so threatened by the actuality of his situation that he retreats into an inner world of fantasy. The patient may use withdrawal as a means of coping with inner anxiety. He may avoid relationships because he anticipates the failure or rejection that he has experienced in past relationships perhaps with those closest to him.

(a) Thought disorder

The patient may be unable to put his thoughts together with clarity and there may be a vagueness or woolliness about his conversation. Concrete thinking may replace the patient's ability to think abstractly and thought blocking may be apparent when the patient begins to talk but stops in mid sentence as if his thoughts have been interrupted. There may be a gap of seconds or several minutes before he resumes the conversation, when he may continue on the same topic or change to a different theme entirely. This loss of thoughts may convince the patient that his thoughts are being stolen (thought withdrawal) or he may believe unwanted thoughts are being placed in his mind (thought insertion). These ideas are evidence of his delusional thinking. At other times the patient may hear his thoughts being broadcast aloud for all to hear. He may engage in the use of new words that he has invented (neologisms). These words have a special meaning which is only known to the patient. In more extreme cases, speech may be totally incoherent and incomprehensible.

(b) Disorders of emotion

At the onset of the illness the patient is often confused and perplexed by his feelings. There is a considerable flattening of affect, so that the patient shows little emotional response to the events occurring around him, or his response may be inappropriate (emotional incongruity). For example he may witness a tragic event with fatuous laughter.

(c) Disturbance of ego function

The development of the ego gives each individual a sense of personal identity. The patient who retreats from reality may have difficulty in distinguishing self from non-self. He may feel dissociated from his own body and from the outside world (depersonalisation). His altered self-perception may account for the long hours he spends gazing in a mirror, as he tries to identify the boundaries of his body.

(d) Withdrawal from reality

The withdrawn patient retreats more and more into his self. He makes no attempt to form relationships with others. He substitutes a world of fantasy for the real world.

(e) Disturbed perception

Hallucinations are false sensory perceptions without any external stimulus. They indicate a break with reality, and are therefore a feature of psychotic illness. There are some exceptions to this rule as hallucinations can occur in normal people under certain conditions, i.e. as a result of sensory deprivation; severe exhaustion; when a person is either falling asleep or waking up (the twilight stages of sleep); or as a result of cortical lesions. Hallucinations can affect any of the five senses.

1 Auditory hallucinations

Auditory hallucinations can range from noises in the head to clear voices which give the patient commands or a running commentary on his actions. Some patients hear themselves being discussed in the third person. Patients react differently to voices and while some seem relatively 'attached' to their voices, others find them distressing, particularly when they are abusive or derogatory. Not all patients will admit to hearing voices and in some instances this can only be assumed because of the patient's behaviour.

2 Visual hallucinations

The patient sees things which are not present in reality. These visions may take the form of flashing lights, geometric patterns, people, animals and objects. Visual hallucinations are common in acute organic states.

3 Tactile hallucinations

Sensations are felt on the surface of the skin or internally. Hallucinatory sensations of a sexual nature may result in complaints of rape or sexual abuse by the patient.

4 Olfactory and gustatory hallucinations

These are hallucinations of smell and taste. Hallucinations of smell are typically associated with the aura in temporal lobe epilepsy. Hallucinations of taste may be associated with beliefs about poisoning.

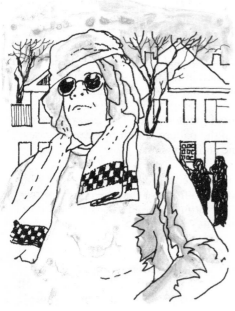

Patient profile

John Wright, aged 19, was a shy and solitary young man. During his first vacation from university, where he was reading history, he announced that he was giving up his studies. His mother tried to get him to discuss his plans for the future, but he appeared to 'switch off' when she tried to talk to him. Over the next few weeks John seemed to become increasingly vague. He was reluctant to get up in the mornings; sometimes he wouldn't get up until tea-time when his father came home.

His behaviour was decidedly odd. On the rare occasions he went out he wore dark glasses (even on the dullest days) and covered his head with several scarves to form a sort of turban. Most of his time was spent in his room where he could be heard engaged in conversation, although there was nobody with him. This was often followed by volatile laughter.

John's mother knew he must be sick, but she didn't approach a doctor for several months. She tried to convince herself that John was just going through a difficult period. She made excuses not to invite friends to the house and she explained John's odd headgear to the neighbours by saying he was suffering

ASSESSMENT INTERVIEW

(Fill in or delete, as appropriate)

Consultant _Dr Issacs_

GP _Dr Fields_

Referred by _GP_

Date of referral _____ Date of admission _10.8.83_

Short-stay ward _Neville Ward_

Medium-stay ward _____

Long-stay ward _____

Day hospital _____

Community Nursing Service _____

Status _Informal_

Surname Mr/~~Mrs/Miss~~ _Wright_

Forenames _John Stuart_

Address _58 Mill Street, Raylton_

Tel. No. _None_

Name of next of kin _Mr and Mrs Wright_

Address _As above_

Tel. No. _None_

Name by which the patient likes to be addressed _John_

Birthday _12.10.61_

DESCRIPTION OF THE PATIENT

Colour of eyes _Blue_   Hair colour _Dark Brown_

Height (m) _1.778_   Weight (kg) _69.9_

Distinguishing features

Sallow complexion, receding hair line. Wears glasses

Present occupation/Occupational history

University Student, dropped out after first term.
Now unemployed

Hobbies and interests

Stamp collecting, modelling toy soldiers, hill walking

Family or persons of significance in patient's life

Mr and Mrs Wright, parents

Persons expected to visit/Support systems

Parents

Religion

Church of England

Home conditions

Lives with parents in terraced house, Raylton, a two bedroomed house recently modernised.

Community services involved/referred

Name of person _Mrs George_

Status _Community Psychiatric Nurse_

Tel. No. _Ext 3330_

Whether contacted (and reason for contacting, if relevant)

To establish a relationship with John prior to his discharge

Psychiatric Condition

Previous psychiatric illness

None

Present psychiatric condition

General appearance _Unshaven, untidily dressed. Mother reports that John covers his head with several scarves if he goes out_

Behaviour _Avoids eye contact. Sits alone, head lowered. Poor response to attempts by nurses to communicate with patient. Appears to be auditory hallucinated - adopts listening posture. Responds to his fantasies by giggling_

Speech patterns/content _Evidence of thought blocking - pauses in mid-sentence then carries on with unrelated topic. Words meaningless when he responds to a question_

Mood _Flattening of affect. Emotional incongruity (inappropriate affect), displayed laughter when he heard that the family cat had been run over_

Orientation _Sometimes, appears to be oblivious to his surroundings, other times confused and perplexed_

Patient's understanding of illness _Difficult to determine at present_

Patient's family's attitudes to patient's illness _Mother is observed to dominate the family. Has her own theories as to the cause of John's behaviour_

61

Present Physical Condition

Result of physical examination

Satisfactory. No abnormalities apparent

Any physical condition for which the patient is receiving treatment?

None

Activities for daily living

Nutrition

Appetite *Fairly good*

Special diet/preferences *eats everything*

Amount of fluid per day *1½ – 2 litres*

Fluid preferences *Tea / Fruit juices*

Elimination

Bowel activity *Regular*

Bladder habit *Normal habit*

Hygiene

Dentures *None*

Washing   Bathing   Dressing
Supervision required with these activities

Mobility and safety factors

Vision *Shortsighted, wears spectacles*

Hearing *Auditory hallucinations*

Sleep patterns *Sleeps soundly*

Menstrual cycle *N/A*

Areas of concern to the patient (list numerically)

Too withdrawn and preoccupied with fantasy to establish

Patient's problems identified during interview (list numerically)

1. Withdrawal from reality.
2. Communicates poorly and inappropriately.
3. Feelings of depersonalisation.
4. Delusions and hallucinations.
5. Apathy.
6. Neglect of personal hygiene.

---

from an ear complaint. John's father kept a low profile in the home, he blamed his wife for John's present state, saying that she had ruined him by her overprotective attitude. The Wrights had not enjoyed a particularly happy marriage, but they managed to 'keep up appearances'. It was Mr Wright who eventually approached the GP. John was admitted to hospital with a schizophrenic illness.

Plan

1. To prevent alienation from human contact.
2. To establish a one to one relationship.
3. To promote an integrated identity.
4. To direct the patient's attention towards reality.
5. To gradually introduce John to ward activities.
6. To encourage a self-care programme.
7. To prevent institutionalisation.
8. To help the patient's family come to terms with his illness.
9. To attend the rehabilitation workshop with a view to obtaining suitable employment.

Implementation

John sat alone absorbed in his world of fantasy, it was the nurse's task to prevent his estrangement from the real world. When trying to establish a relationship with John a one-to-one approach was found to be best. John may have felt threatened by the presence of several nurses.

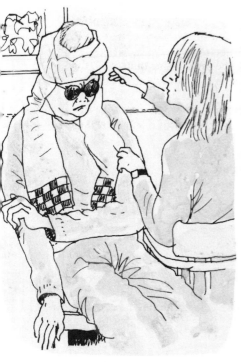

One nurse was allocated to spend some time with him each day; she sat beside him, occasionally talking to him about general topics. It was difficult for the nurse to communicate with John, and it involved a special effort on her part. Argyle and Trower[1] write that poor communications are seen by others as unrewarding because they fail to respond or give feedback.

The nurse had to learn to accept her own feelings of anxiety during the long periods of silence. By being with John she communicated the concern of one human being for another.

The nurse discovered from John's mother that he liked modelling and painting, although he had done neither recently. She tried to recreate his interest by providing him with the necessary materials. This proved to be the first medium through which John was able to express his feelings, and allowed the staff to view John's world as he perceived it.

After several weeks in the ward John began to respond verbally to the nurse's efforts to communicate with him. He said 'I am an alien from another planet. . . my body is an empty shell'. . ., the nurse listened to John's conversation to establish the complexity of his delusional thinking. She never reinforced his delusions or tried to argue with him.

When John appeared to be listening to voices, the nurse observed the effects on his behaviour, i.e. whether he became distressed or excitable. She was aware that voices sometimes command patients to harm others and can account for unpredictable attacks of violence. The nurse recorded her observations in the Kardex, as accurately as possible, writing down what John said. When caring for a patient who is deluded or hallucinated the nurse found the best approach was to care for the person without supporting his symptoms of illness. The nurse promoted John's integrated identity by accepting him as an individual and helping him to be accepted by others. Being preoccupied with his inner world John tended to neglect his personal hygiene. He had to be encouraged to engage in self-care activities by gentle coaxing.

John met his dietary needs adequately, although some withdrawn patients require assistance with feeding. His nursing care included the giving of prescribed medication, observing and reporting any side effects.

After six weeks in hospital John was able to participate in a wider range of activities. He was able to leave the ward without his headgear. He spent several weekends at home, and was eventually well enough to live at home while attending the Rehabilitation Unit. He enjoyed the tasks he was given, although his work output was slow. John lacked initiative, and still tended to avoid eye contact. He had no desire to return to university, and no goals for the future. When John's parents were seen by the doctor they admitted that there was considerable conflict in their marriage, but declined the offer to participate in family therapy, therefore it was impossible to help the family as a unit.

Rationale

Much of the improvement in the treatment of schizophrenia has been attributed to the nurse's relationship with the patient.

Evaluation

John's progress was slow. Several of the nurses managed to establish a relationship with him; although John seemed to like these particular nurses he rarely initiated any conversation with them.

As John became less withdrawn he gradually became more willing to take responsibility for his own self-care. His delusions and hallucinations were no longer evident and he spent several weekends at home.

John eventually became well enough to attend the Rehabilitation Centre. At first he attended from the ward; later he was discharged and attended the centre daily from home.

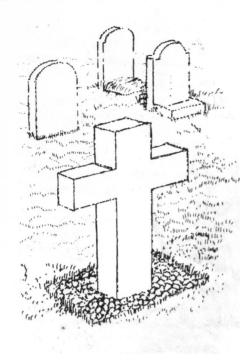

Mrs George, the Community Psychiatric Nurse, had established rapport with John while he was in hospital, and continued to visit him at the Rehabilitation Centre and gave him his Depixol injections.

John enjoyed the work and seemed to be progressing quite well, then without warning he committed suicide. He gave no clues to others of his intentions and had not appeared to be depressed.

Assessing the suicidal risk in patients suffering from schizophrenia can be difficult. Morgan[2] suggests that a high proportion of unexpected suicides may be due to this condition.

John had difficulty in expressing his innermost self to others and sadly this prevented others from reaching out to him.

John's parents were visited by the Community Psychiatric Nurse who offered her support in their bereavement.

References

1. Argyle, M. and Trower, P., *Person to Person — Ways of Communicating*, Life Cycle Books, 1980
2. Morgan, H.G., *Death Wishes — The Understanding and Management of Deliberate Self Harm*, Wiley, 1979

Chapter 8

Nursing the patient who is suspicious

Introduction

When a person experiences feelings of paranoia he is convinced that others are acting against him in an unfriendly way. Most people can recall having such feelings on occasions in response to everyday events. In the patient suffering from a paranoid reaction such feelings form a predominant part of his personality.

The individual is usually highly sensitive and easily offended. He is suspicious about the motives of others, and consequently has few friends. Isolation caused by deafness or physical illness can sometimes be a precipitating factor.

Paranoid states have a gradual onset usually developing after the age of 40. The person may think that the remarks people make, or actions of people he meets, have some special significance for him. This is called Ideas of Reference. When delusional thinking develops, the patient is able to cover this well at first; his personality is well preserved and he is able to give a coherent account of his false beliefs.

It is often difficult to pinpoint where normality ends and delusional thinking begins. Because the patient's beliefs seem so real and convincing, sometimes another person, usually a close relative, can also perceive the evironment as being hostile. This is called Folie à Deux. Paranoid states are often difficult to treat because of the patient's ability to hide his illness for a considerable time before it is recognised.

Paranoid delusions may also be a feature of schizophrenia, organic states and affective disorders.

Patient profile

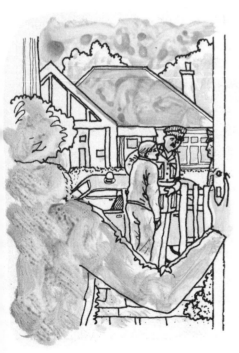

Jack Smithfield, aged 59, was a farm labourer/handyman on a large estate, where he occupied one of the estate's cottages. He was a quiet, reserved person who enjoyed the outdoor life. He had no family as his parents had died several years ago and his only brother had been killed in rather tragic circumstances when they were both children.

Jack kept very much to himself. He never married because he'd stayed at home to care for his parents after they retired from service up at the manor. His only companion was his dog Paddy, who virtually went everywhere with him.

One evening in late summer, when the haymaking was over Jack walked purposefully down to the village calling at the home of Mrs Brew, a widow in her 70s. He told her he'd come about the house. He wanted to know when she was leaving. The old lady, who only knew Jack by sight, explained that there must be some misunderstanding as she had no intention of leaving; Jack muttered something and walked away.

A few weeks later Jack called on Mrs Brew again; this time his manner was aggressive, he said he wanted her out of his house by the end of the week because he was going to move in. The old lady was frightened and shut her door quickly; Jack continued to shout and threaten her through the letter box.

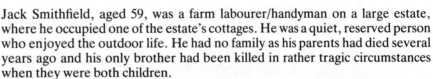

The police were called and Jack was admitted to hospital under section 136 of the Mental Health Act 1983. Having no next of kin his employer was informed of the evening's events, and he agreed to make arrangements for Jack's dog to be looked after whilst Jack was in hospital.

ASSESSMENT INTERVIEW

(Fill in or delete, as appropriate)

Consultant _Dr Sands_

GP _Dr Glover_

Referred by _____

Date of referral _____ Date of admission _20.7.83_

Short-stay ward _Neville Ward_

Medium-stay ward _____

Long-stay ward _____

Day hospital _____

Community Nursing Service _✓_

Status _Section 136_

Surname Mr/~~Mrs/Miss~~ _Smithfield_

Forenames _Jack Arthur_

Address _No. 6, Estate Cottages,_
The Manor, Raylton

Tel. No. _None_

Name of next of kin _Mr Fenton Brown, Employer_

Address _The Manor, Raylton_

Tel. No. _01 060 6669_

Name by which the patient likes to be addressed _Jack_

Birthday _3.1.21_

DESCRIPTION OF THE PATIENT

Colour of eyes _Grey/Blue_ Hair colour _Grey_

Height (m) _1.778_ Weight (kg) _73.0_

Distinguishing features
Ruddy complexion, curly mop of
grey hair, bushy eyebrows

Present occupation/Occupational history
Farm labourer and general handyman
on large estate, was born on estate
and has only worked for the one family
all his life

Hobbies and interests
Following local hunt, works as a beater
when shoots are held on estate.
Wood carving

Family or persons of significance in patient's life
No family. Parents dead. A younger
brother was killed in a shooting
accident at the age of nine

Persons expected to visit/Support systems
Not known

Religion
Methodist

Home conditions
Small cottage on estate. Sparsely
furnished but spotlessly clean

Community services involved/referred
Name of person _Mr Paul Scott_

Status _Community Psychiatric Nurse_

Tel. No. _Ext 7142_

Whether contacted (and reason for contacting, if relevant)
Yes

Psychiatric Condition

Previous psychiatric illness
None. Father was a heavy drinker.
Mother suffered a depressive
illness after Jack was born

Present psychiatric condition

General appearance _A well-nourished man with_
a ruddy complexion

Behaviour _Smokes occasionally_
Tense in company

Speech patterns/content _Expresses delusional_
beliefs - thinks he owns a house in
the village. Swears at nurses when
approached

Mood _Generally quiet, withdrawn and_
suspicious

Orientation _Normal_

Patient's understanding of illness _He has no_
insight into illness

Patient's family's attitudes to patient's illness _____
No family

Present Physical Condition

Result of physical examination

Slight deafness—to be referred to ENT consultant. Smokes about 15 cigarettes a day

Any physical condition for which the patient is receiving treatment?

Deafness to be investigated, appointment obtained for 2 weeks' time

Activities for daily living

Nutrition

Appetite _Moderate_

Special diet/preferences _Lots of fresh vegetables_

Amount of fluid per day _2 litres_

Fluid preferences _Milk, doesn't drink tea_

Elimination

Bowel activity _Regular_

Bladder habit _Normal_

Hygiene

Dentures _None_

Washing Bathing Dressing

Minimal supervision required with these activities

Mobility and safety factors

Vision _Normal_

Hearing _Deafness_

Sleep patterns _Sleeps soundly_

Menstrual cycle _N/A_

Areas of concern to the patient (list numerically)

Patient is convinced that his dog has been put down, and that he will be turned out of his cottage.

Patient's problems identified during interview (list numerically)

1. Suspiciousness.
2. Avoids company.
3. Deafness.
4. Delusional thinking. Believes his dog has been destroyed (despite being told otherwise) and that he will be forced to leave his tied cottage.

Plan

1. To establish a relationship with the patient.
2. To communicate clearly with the patient because of his deafness.
3. To develop areas of his personality untouched by delusional thinking.
4. To arrange for the patient to see his dog.
5. To establish rapport with the Community Psychiatric Nurse, who will be responsible for giving the patient his medication before and after discharge.

Implementation

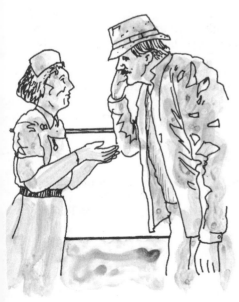

When trying to establish a relationship with Jack the nurse took particular care to be honest and truthful in her dealings with him. She never appeared to pry into his background or affairs, or isolate him because he was hostile and rejecting.

Crawford and Buchanan[1] suggest that the nurse should accept the patient's rebuffs and abusive language as symptoms of his illness and not as personal attacks.

Lancaster[2] describes the primary objective of nursing intervention as creating a safe and trusting relationship with the patient, so that he can forfeit some of his psychological isolation. It was only when he was able to recognise the consistent qualities of the nurse that a trusting relationship began to develop. Jack was given as much freedom as possible; restrictions would only reinforce his feelings that people were against him. He was never forced into group activities against his will and because he felt others undermined him was given the responsibility of checking the weekly stores.

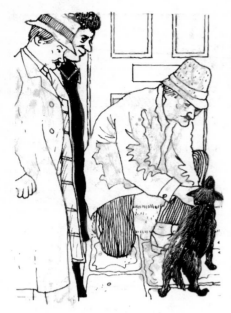

Deafness is known to contribute towards feelings of isolation and may be a causative factor in the development of paranoid thinking. When addressing Jack the nurse spoke clearly and directly to him, using words that were familiar and easily understood. Talking away from him would only increase his suspiciousness. The nurse ensured that all members of the team were aware of the patient's hearing difficulty. She exercised care in the use of non-verbal communication when addressing Jack, did not smile too freely or touch him in case this should arouse his suspicions about her motives for trying to befriend him.

Another problem that arose was that Jack refused to take his medication. It took some time for the nurse to convince him that the drugs would aid his recovery. She knew that if she hid his tablets in his food she could lose what trust she had gained altogether.

When delusional beliefs were expressed the nurse didn't argue with Jack as this would only serve to convince him that he was not understood, and he might then put up further barriers between himself and others. The nurse found it was better to listen passively, neither agreeing or disagreeing, to what he had to say. The content of Jack's delusional thinking expressed in his conversation was accurately recorded in the Kardex, as delusions concerning other patients and staff could lead to violent behaviour.

The nurse tried to develop areas of the patient's personality untouched by delusional thinking by encouraging him to expand his interests and skills through involvement in ward activities and occupational therapy.

The Community Psychiatric Nurse was invited to establish rapport with Jack and to commence giving him his injections of Modecate, as these injections were to be continued after his discharge. The patient who is suspicious is more likely to consent to continued medication from a nurse who has been able to develop a relationship with him during his hospitalisation.

Rationale

Consistent honesty helps to reduce the patient's doubts about others.

Evaluation

It was not easy to establish a relationship with Jack at first, but the nurses persevered in a matter-of-fact way without making the patient feel stifled.

An important factor in Jack's case was the discovery of his hearing difficulties, and arranging for him to be fitted with a suitable aid. Once Jack became accustomed to the appliance, he seemed to be happier and less suspicious.

The Community Psychiatric Nurse gave Jack his Modecate injections during his hospitalisation. An important factor in Jack's agreement to continue the injections when discharged was the nurse's relationship with him. However several months after leaving hospital Jack refused to have any more injections saying he disliked needles.

Despite this Jack remained well, kept his out-patient appointments and maintained a relationship with the Community Psychiatric Nurse who continues to visit him.

References

1. Crawford, A.L. and Buchanan, B.B., *Psychiatric Nursing. A Basic Manual,* Davis, 1961
2. Lancaster, J., *Adult Psychiatric Nursing,* Medical Examination Publishing Co., 1980

Chapter 9

Nursing the patient who is aggressive

Introduction

Aggression is a normal drive. Much of Man's aggression is released through his work and leisure activities. Aggression ranges along a continuum from sullen, resentful and hostile behaviour to forms of verbal expression and violent acts involving physical force.

Although we live in a society where violence is ever present, aggression always presents problems for the nurse caring for the mentally ill. Such behaviour may occur among patients suffering from delusions and hallucinations or among confused patients who misinterpret their surroundings.

There are some individuals who have not learned to express their aggressive energy through appropriate channels of expression. Folkard[2] states that aggression may become an individual's habitual mode of behaviour in certain situations in an attempt to gain goals or rewards. This applies to the psychopathic personality, who is unable to postpone gratification and will obtain his goals come what may; his poorly developed super-ego prevents him from experiencing guilt or remorse for his misdeeds.

The nurse may encounter a patient with a psychopathic personality; he is a plausible individual who may exhibit a superficial charm on first acquaintance, is insincere and unable to form close relationships. Nevertheless he is skilful in blaming others for his own mistakes. His impulsive and anti-social acts cause problems not only for himself but also for society.

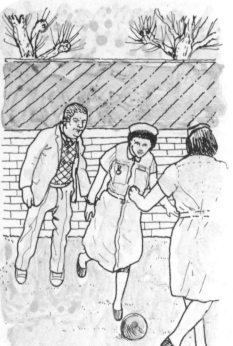

Patient profile

Charlie, the youngest of three boys, was eight when his father walked out on the family. His mother worked hard to bring up the children, but found three boys difficult to manage without male support. She disliked arguments and gave in to her children's demands for the sake of peace. Charlie didn't like school and his rebellious behaviour got him into trouble on many occasions. He was unable to learn from his mistakes. Throughout his early schooling he was often away with minor complaints; later, he played truant and attempted to cover his absence with notes purporting to come from his mother; he felt no remorse when found out. Despite his poor schooling attendance, Charlie had no difficulty in obtaining jobs. At interviews, he came across as an intelligent and articulate young man. This plausibility convinced prospective employers that he was more than suitable. But Charlie lacked perseverance, routine bored him; he never remained in any job for long. His restless and impulsive nature led him to seek greener pastures.

Charlie's last job was as a sales representative, and he had made a very favourable impression on his employers in the short time he had been with them. However, he was instantly dismissed after a minor disagreement during which he punched one of the directors. Charlie couldn't tolerate frustration; he reacted in the only way he knew how — by lashing out.

Shortly after this, Charlie's girlfriend, with whom he had been living for three months, threw him out and he took an overdose of aspirin. He was treated at his local hospital and referred to a psychiatrist. Dr Sands decided to admit him to the unit, because he appeared to be depressed.

ASSESSMENT INTERVIEW

(Fill in or delete, as appropriate)

Consultant _Dr Sands_

GP _Dr Evans_

Referred by _Dr Sands_

Date of referral _____ Date of admission _25.8.83_

Short-stay ward _Reynolds_

Medium-stay ward _____

Long-stay ward _____

Day hospital _____

Community Nursing Service _____

Status _Informal_

Surname Mr/~~Mrs/Miss~~ _Ross_

Forenames _Charles John_

Address _99 Queens Parkway, Raylton_

Tel. No. _01 003 2515_

Name of next of kin _Mrs A Ross_ Relationship _mother_

Address _As above_

Tel. No. _____

Name by which the patient likes to be addressed _Charlie_

Birthday _14.2.62_

DESCRIPTION OF THE PATIENT

Colour of eyes _Blue_   Hair colour _Blond_

Height (m) _1.753_   Weight (kg) _69.8_

Distinguishing features
Dark complexion, well groomed. Small scar left side of chin

Present occupation/Occupational history
Eight different jobs since leaving school in 1978, all in a selling capacity. Most recent sales representative, double glazing. Unemployed one month

Hobbies and interests
Mainly opposite sex, football, cinema, dancing

Family or persons of significance in patient's life
Mrs A Ross, mother

Persons expected to visit/Support systems
Mother and brothers

Religion
None

Home conditions
Shared rented flat with girlfriend until thrown out, moved back home temporarily

Community services involved/referred

Name of person _None_

Status _____

Tel. No. _____

Whether contacted (and reason for contacting, if relevant)

_____

Psychiatric Condition

Previous psychiatric illness
No previous history

Present psychiatric condition

General appearance _A presentable young man, calm and responsive_

Behaviour _sociable, mixes well_

Speech patterns/content _Talks willingly, no hesitancy_

Mood _No marked depression apparent_

Orientation _Within normal boundaries_

Patient's understanding of illness _Gives the impression that he understands the reasons for his admission but appears to lack any genuine insight_

Patient's family's attitudes to patient's illness _Mother shows a negative response to her son's well being_

Present Physical Condition

Result of physical examination

General health good

Any physical condition for which the patient is receiving treatment?

None

Activities for daily living

Nutrition

Appetite _____ _Good_

Special diet/preferences _Steak and chips_

Amount of fluid per day _2½ litres_

Fluid preferences _____ _Beer_

Elimination

Bowel activity _Regular pattern_

Bladder habit _Normal habit_

Hygiene

Dentures _____ _None_

Washing Bathing Dressing

No assistance required

Mobility and safety factors

Vision _____ _Good_

Hearing _____ _Good_

Sleep patterns _Sleeps well_

Menstrual cycle _____ _N/A_

Areas of concern to the patient (list numerically)

Feels a sense of failure, says he has achieved nothing of consequence in his life

Patient's problems identified during interview (list numerically)

1. The patient's low tolerance for frustration may lead to violent outbursts.

2. Is able to detect areas of discontent among others and manipulate relationships to cause further upset.

3. The patient has expressed suicidal intent.

4. His sense of failure.

Plan

1. To prevent violent behaviour by encouraging the patient to express his aggressive drive in socially acceptable ways.
2. To minimise factors which may potentiate violent behaviour.
3. To ensure that all staff are familiar with local policy for dealing with violent incidents.
4. To adopt an open and honest approach towards the patient in an attempt to reduce his opportunities for manipulative behaviour.
5. To assist the patient to establish some long-term goals.
6. To prevent suicide.

Implementation

Charlie was diagnosed as suffering from a psychopathic personality. Being unable to tolerate frustration he presented a potential risk with regard to aggressive behaviour. It was the nurse's task to help Charlie learn new and socially acceptable ways of expressing his anger. He was encouraged to talk about his feelings, as this provided some relief for his inner tension. At this stage the nurse recalled the ways in which she dealt with her own feelings of anger; she usually engaged in some form of physical activity. She found that self-examination enhanced her understanding of the patient's problems.

Charlie was encouraged to release his feelings of anger through a programme of activities which included physical exercise, sport, games and creative hobbies. Actions involving hammering, thumping and tearing were particularly useful.

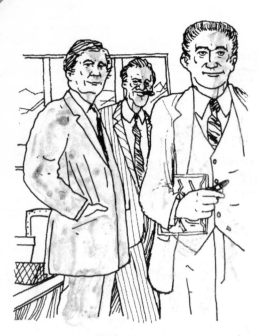

The nurse participated in Charlie's planned activities. This was the best way to develop a relationship and really get to know him as a person. As an active participant, the nurse was more acceptable as a role model. She was also in a better position to observe him for clues which indicated a change of mood. She noted that he became silent and withdrawn when he was feeling tense and avoided eye contact; it was only by really getting to know Charlie well that the nurse was able to recognise these signs. She encouraged him to release his feelings in a mature and appropriate manner. Usually he could be persuaded to sit in a quiet area of the ward and verbalise his feelings. Environmental factors which could serve to potentiate aggressiveness were kept to a minimum; these included unnecessary rules and restrictions, jealousy, fear, overcrowding, provocation by other patients and staff and broken promises.

Despite every attempt by the nursing staff to control the patient's behaviour by the provision of suitable outlets, there was an incident in which Charlie threatened to 'carve up' another patient with a broken bottle. The nurse quietly summoned help and then tried to pacify him tactfully. Other patients were removed or kept away from the incident area for their own safety. The nurse tried to behave in a calm manner, not betraying her own feelings of anxiety in an already highly charged situation. She removed her watch and other items which could harm the patient or be used by him as a weapon. It was necessary to restrain Charlie when he became intent on carrying out his threat to the other patient; he was approached by several nurses who held him firmly by his clothing, avoiding injury to the vulnerable parts of his body. He was taken to the gym where he was encouraged to engage in strenuous physical activity. The incident was reported in the Kardex, and an attempt was made to identify the factors which led up to the incident, although in this case none could be found. The names of the staff who were present and had assisted in restraining Charlie were noted. Fortunately there were no injuries to other patients or staff, and no damage to hospital property.

Castledine[1] suggests that after any violent incident, discussion with the patient should take place to find out what happened and possible alternatives sought, in case such an incident occurs again.

Despite Charlie's superficial charm, he had a great capacity for causing discord among the other patients; he was able to play one individual off against another with considerable ease. He showed no feelings of remorse for the trouble he caused.

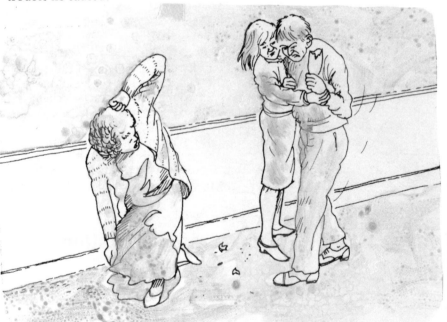

He was not depressed but expressed a sense of failure because he had never achieved anything worthwhile. The possibility remained that Charlie might make a further suicidal attempt and for this reason he was constantly observed.

After several weeks in the ward the Consultant decided that Charlie would benefit more in the long term if cared for in a therapeutic community setting. There he would be taught to accept responsibility for his own actions.

As the hospital did not offer this particular facility arrangements were made for Charlie's transfer to Coombe Wood Hospital in Surrey.

Rationale

By helping the aggressive patient to release his inner tension through socially acceptable channels, it protects the patient himself and others from the harmful consequences of his aggression.

Evaluation

Charlie was admitted because he had appeared to be depressed after making a suicide attempt. He showed no signs of depression or any evidence of suicidal intention while under continuous observation. Charlie's aggressive behaviour placed other patients at risk; the nurses assisted him to channel this aggressive energy into socially acceptable activities and attempted to reduce potentiating factors to a minimum.

The senior nurse ensured that all the staff were familiar with the hospital policy for dealing with incidents of violent and aggressive behaviour.

The decision to send Charlie to a therapeutic community was reached in order to maintain a safe environment for the other patients and to enable the patient to be treated in a milieu that would promote more positive and lasting changes in his behaviour.

The nurses would be very sorry to see Charlie go — when he was nice he was very nice!

The therapeutic milieu

This refers to the patient's environment which is utilised in a positive way to enable him to learn new and more fulfilling patterns of behaviour.

Fact sheet: When a patient is violent

There are times when, despite the nurse's efforts, a patient does behave violently. The following are guidelines to the action that should be taken:

1. Try to pacify the patient using as much tact as possible. Bear in mind that he will often respond to a nurse who has established a good relationship with him.
2. Keep other patients away for their own safety.
3. Behave in a calm manner and do not over-react in an already highly charged tense situation.
4. Never tackle the patient alone, and avoid being cornered by the patient.
5. Summon help. The presence of a number of staff may deter the patient.
6. Never forget that the patient is ill and must be protected.
7. Avoid injury to the patient, other patients and staff if physical restraint of the patient becomes necessary.
8. Remove any items which could damage the patient or could be damaged by the patient, e.g. spectacles, rings, watches or any object that could be used as a weapon.
9. If the patient must be restrained, hold his clothing rather than his body, avoid any pressure on vulnerable areas such as his head, throat, chest, abdomen and pelvis, or fingers.

Fact sheet: Reporting incidents of violence

The report should cover:

1. The patient's behaviour which led up to the outburst.
2. Identification of any factors leading up to the incident if this is possible.
3. An accurate objective report of the action which was taken and the names of the staff who assisted in restraining the patient.
4. Injuries to the patient or others.
5. Damage to personal or hospital property.

The report should be submitted to the Senior Nurse Manager. The nurse should be directed by the local guidelines of her own health authority on dealing with aggression or violence.

Fact sheet: Prevention of violent behaviour

Violent and impulsive behaviour can often be prevented if the nurse:

1. Gets to know the patient well as a person.
2. Provides activities which allow the patient to release natural aggressive energy in socially acceptable ways.
3. Is honest in her dealings with the patient.
4. Reduces factors within the patient's environment which may potentiate violent behaviour. Examples of these factors are as follows: overcrowding, broken promises, jealousy, lack of privacy, restricted freedom, fear, apprehension, frustration, boredom, provocation by staff and other patients, arguments and lack of respect.

Fact sheet: A therapeutic community

This type of approach provides patients with an environment structured in such a way that it promotes positive changes in their behaviour. The therapeutic environment encourages self-expression and uses group processes as its main tool in restoring mental homeostasis.

Among patients who benefit from this type of approach are the psychopathic personalities who have difficulty in controlling their aggressive impulses. Such patients are subjected to peer group pressure and are accountable to the group for their behaviour. Thus behaviour which fails to comply to the group's norms and values is met by group confrontation; group cohesiveness is such that it will not allow its members to be endangered by threatening or destructive behaviour. The patient who engages in anti-social behaviour learns to accept responsibility for his actions; failure to conform can result in isolation from the group.

Nursing staff play a minimal role in comparison to more traditional psychiatric nursing. They wear no uniform to identify themselves. They actively encourage patient autonomy and independence. The patients take responsibilities for day to day running of the ward and problems are discussed at daily meetings.

Both staff and patients are committed to the overall philosophy of the therapeutic community. Group influence is a powerful force in the control of harmful and undesirable behaviour. It allows new learning to take place and has a more effective therapeutic value in behavioural change than standards imposed on the patient by nursing staff.

References

1. Castledine, G., *Nursing Mirror*, **153**, 12, September 16, 1981
2. Folkard, M.S., *A Sociological Contribution to the Understanding of Aggression and its Treatment,* Netherne Hospital Press, 1957

Chapter 10

Nursing the patient who is confused

Introduction

The confused patient usually conveys this from his behaviour: he looks bewildered and is slow to comprehend what is happening around him. He is unable to express himself coherently and may be disorientated, not knowing who he is, where he is or what day it is. The periods of confusion may alternate with phases of lucidity.

In the general hospital the nurse will have met patients who are confused following head injuries or post-operatively; she may have nursed patients suffering from severe anaemia, cardiac or renal failure and observed evidence of confused behaviour.

In the psychiatric hospital the nurse may encounter anxious or depressed patients who complain of feeling confused, but more frequently will be called upon to care for elderly patients throughout many different fields of nursing.

In some individuals mental deterioration precedes any physical changes; when other causes have been eliminated these patients may be suffering from the irreversible changes of senile dementia. These changes in the brain lead to progressive mental deterioration. One of the most striking changes is the patient's impairment of memory; recent happenings are forgotten while events of long ago are recalled easily. Sometimes a person is aware of his difficulties and begins to run his life to a strict routine. He makes out long lists of what he has to do, and may unconsciously attempt to fill in his memory gaps by telling stories or confabulating.

As the illness progresses the patient's orientation becomes more impaired and it may be distressing for his family when he fails to recognise them. Uninhibited and anti-social behaviour can occur when brain damage results in the lifting of normal social constraints.

Self-care is neglected and decreasing intellectual functioning impairs judgement, understanding and the recall of knowledge. The individual may show increasing stubbornness, belligerence, and insusceptibility to change.

Fish[2] suggests that personality traits tend to be enhanced by ageing, but the only personality change which is always associated with ageing is rigidity.

There may be rapid spontaneous variations in emotional response and the individual may weep easily.

Confusion and restlessness may be worse at night; the patient may wander through the streets purposelessly, being susceptible to many dangers.

There is no cure for the condition of senile dementia, but the quality of the patient's life can be enhanced through skilled nursing care.

Whitehead[4] writes that half the beds for the mentally ill in this country are occupied by old people. They have got into such accommodation either because they have developed illnesses in their youth, which have kept them in hospital ever since, or they have become mentally ill in old age.

The nurse will therefore encounter many elderly patients in a psychiatric hospital who will benefit from the process of nursing.

Patient profile

Mrs Galbraith, aged 70, had lived in Raylton with her husband for the past four years. Their old home in Barnford had been demolished to make way for a new shopping complex. Both had adapted well to the change. They had three sons and a daughter, all married; the eleven grandchildren were Mr and Mrs Galbraith's pride and joy.

ASSESSMENT INTERVIEW

(Fill in or delete, as appropriate)

Consultant _Dr Lyle_
GP _Dr Irons_
Referred by _GP_
Date of referral _____ Date of admission _2.2.83_
Short-stay ward _____
Medium-stay ward _____
Long-stay ward _Russell_
Day hospital _____
Community Nursing Service _District Nurse_
Status _____

Surname ~~Mr/Mrs/Miss~~ _Galbraith_
Forenames _Annie Dorothy_
Address _14 Willow Court, New Raylton_
_____

Tel. No. _7600 (daughter)_
Name of next of kin _Mr Arthur Galbraith Husband_
Address _As above_
_____

Tel. No. _____
Name by which the patient likes to be addressed _Mrs Galbraith_
Birthday _12.6.11_

DESCRIPTION OF THE PATIENT
Colour of eyes _Blue_   Hair colour _Silver Grey_
Height (m) _1.473_   Weight (kg) _44.5_

Distinguishing features
Small, frail lady, thinning hair
_____

Present occupation/Occupational history
Housewife / seamstress before
retirement

Hobbies and interests
Cooking, sewing, knitting, television
_____

Family or persons of significance in patient's life
Husband, Mr Arthur Galbraith, daughter,
Mrs Sylvia Day and her family her three
sons and daughter-in-law Eleven grandchildren
Persons expected to visit/Support systems
Husband in hospital at present
Her children and their families
Religion
Church of England

Home conditions
Two bedroomed ground floor flat in
a small block of 18
_____

Community services involved/referred
Name of person _Mrs Brewer_
Status _District Nurse_
Tel. No. _1144_
Whether contacted (and reason for contacting, if relevant)
Yes

Psychiatric Condition

Previous psychiatric illness
None, but has been becoming
increasing forgetful for a number
of years

Present psychiatric condition
General appearance _Small frail lady, posture_
good, who appears bewildered

Behaviour _Periods of anxiety, attention_
and judgement impaired

Speech patterns/content _Talks about events of_
her past life, but unable to recall
recent events and happenings.
Uses words inaccurately. Confabulates,
answers questions other than the ones
asked. Conversation repetitious

Mood _Mood changes rapidly, easily moved_
to tears

Orientation _Disorientated, unable to recall_
where she is, but calls the nurses by
her daughter's name - Sylvia. Doesn't
always answer to her own name

Patient's understanding of illness _During lucid_
intervals may have some insight, but
unable to say why she was in
hospital

Patient's family's attitudes to patient's illness _Accept need_
for hospitalisation on a temporary
basis until husband is discharged
from hospital

Present Physical Condition

Result of physical examination

Mild cardiac failure. Ankle and sacral oedema

Any physical condition for which the patient is receiving treatment?

Cardiac failure and oedema

Activities for daily living

Nutrition

Appetite _Needs encouragement and supervision with diet_

Special diet/preferences _Will need a soft diet_

Amount of fluid per day _1½ litres   Encourage fluids_

Fluid preferences _Likes blackcurrant drinks_

Elimination

Bowel activity _Constipation_

Bladder habit _Incontinent_

Hygiene

Dentures _Refuses to wear them_

Washing   Bathing   Dressing

Needs assistance in all these areas

Mobility and safety factors

Vision _Glasses for reading_

Hearing _Slight deafness_

Sleep patterns _Confusion and disorientation worse at night_

Menstrual cycle _Not relevant_

Areas of concern to the patient (list numerically)

In lucid intervals asks 'Why isn't Arthur here?'

Patient's problems identified during interview (list numerically)

1. A loss of identity, i.e. she doesn't always know who she is.
2. The environment may pose threats to her safety.
3. She is unable to meet her basic needs without assistance.
4. She requires the love and care of her family.
5. She needs to live a regular and ordered life with a balance between activity stimulation and rest.
6. Her lifestyle should be as self-fulfilling as possible.

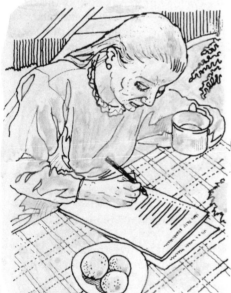

Their daughter, Sylvia, lived locally and called in most days; the sons lived some distance away but visited regularly.

Mrs Galbraith's memory had been bad for some time. She found it necessary to write out long lists of what she had to do. A few weeks prior to her admission to hospital she had put a pan of fat on to the stove to heat up and had forgotten about it. Fortunately Mr Galbraith smelt the fumes, and his quick action prevented a fire. There had been similar incidents over the past year, and Mr Galbraith didn't like his wife being in the kitchen unless he was there.

Sometimes Mrs Galbraith told stories which were totally untrue; her husband found it pointless to argue with her because she would only burst into tears. There were times when she would insist on calling the cat before they

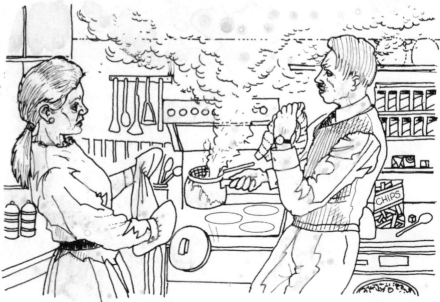

went to bed; the cat had died some years ago and they'd never had another since moving to Willow Court. There were times when Mr Galbraith felt quite embarrassed by his wife's behaviour. Increasingly she became more and more difficult to manage; urinary incontinence became a problem and there was an accident at least once a day because Mrs Galbraith had forgotten where the toilet was. Periods of confusion and perplexity were becoming more apparent and to make matters worse Mr Galbraith found his wife could be very obstinate. Eventually his own health began to suffer; there were times when he felt quite depressed. He was reluctant to go and see his GP 'in case they put Annie away'. Sylvia helped by sleeping at her parents' home two nights per week to enable her father to get some proper rest, but there were limits to what she could do without causing hardship in their own family. Eventually, realising the futility of the situation, she approached the doctor herself.

Respecting Mr Galbraith's wishes to care for his wife at home, the doctor arranged for the district nurse to call, and laundry and home help were also provided. The arrangement worked very well, and Mr Galbraith found it easier to manage his wife between the nurse's visits.

Then Mr Galbraith developed chronic bronchitis and heart failure and had to be admitted to hospital. The GP arranged for Mrs Galbraith to be admitted to the local psychiatric hospital until such time her husband was discharged. Mr Galbraith was in hospital for eight weeks; he responded well to treatment but on discharge was still left with some shortness of breath. His immediate thoughts were for his wife; he wanted her home but neither his GP nor the geriatrician felt that Mr Galbraith could continue to care for his wife even with the additional support he had been receiving. His wife's mental condition had been exacerbated by a respiratory infection; although she recovered from this the periods of confusion became more frequent.

A case conference was held on the ward, Mr Galbraith and his family were invited. The patient's progress and plans for her future were discussed and it was explained to Mr Galbraith and his family that Mrs Galbraith's mental condition would progressively worsen; eventually long-term hospitalisation would almost certainly be necessary. Mr Galbraith's present health status would make it difficult for him to manage his wife at home as she now needed twenty-four hour care.

Mr Galbraith reluctantly agreed with the doctor's proposal, he knew his own health limitations; despite the staff being very kind and showing him and his daughter around the ward, he felt very sad when he went home. He'd promised to love Annie in sickness and in health. Somehow, he felt he'd let her down.

Plan

1. To promote the quality of life through individualised care.
2. To support the patient's family.
3. To preserve the patient's individual identity.
4. To exercise control over Mrs Galbraith's environment in order to promote her safety.
5. To maintain hygiene, physical comfort and freedom from pain. To communicate effectively with the patient.
6. To provide a regular routine in which the patient can live a meaningful life.
7. To prevent environmental deprivation by providing stimulation through the provision of simple activities.
8. To facilitate regular bladder and bowel function.
9. To promote peaceful sleep.
10. To enable the patient to meet her nutritional needs.

Implementation

While it is not possible to reverse the process of dementia much can be achieved through skilled nursing care, improving the quality of the patient's life.

Eliopoulos[1] writes that aged individuals share similar universal self-care demands with all other human beings. A degree of sensitivity and awareness are necessary on the nurse's part to identify Mrs Galbraith's needs; her life was made as fulfilling and normal as possible. Mrs Galbraith was cared for among a small group of patients; one nurse was allocated to their care; another nurse was available to give assistance as necessary. This allowed the nurse to get to know her patients individually and enabled the patients to recognise her as their nurse. It also allowed the more dependent patients to be shared equally among the nurses.

As with her companions, Mrs Galbraith was dressed in her own clothes, and allowed to have some of her personal possessions in her sleeping area. She was encouraged to meet her own self-care needs as far as she was able, in order to preserve her independence. She was always addressed as Mrs Galbraith; endearments were not used as these can be upsetting to patients, and does nothing to reinforce their individuality. The nurse maintained a safe environment for the patient, because Mrs Galbraith was confused, her attention and judgement were impaired, and the nurse had to ensure her safety by reducing environmental hazards. Slippery floors, worn rugs, unstable furniture and poorly lit areas have no place in the geriatric ward.

Sudden movements were avoided; to prevent giddiness when Mrs Galbraith was getting up in the morning or standing up after sitting in a chair, she was helped to change her position gradually to facilitate adaptation. Early detection of any physical signs of illness was essential. Kastenbaum[3] states that a person may not just be senile but disordered in thought and behaviour *because* of undetected or poorly treated illness. Thus the nurse was aware that physical illness could exacerbate the patient's confusion, and reported any changes in the patient's physical condition to the doctor.

Regular chiropody was incorporated into the care programme to ensure that callouses or long nails didn't make walking painful; the nurse ensured that her patient wore well fitting shoes to aid her balance. Communicating with the patient was an essential feature of nursing care. Body language, particularly touch, provided Mrs Galbraith with a sense of reassurance, security and belonging. Non-verbal communication is even more important when there is some degree of sensory impairment.

A regular routine within a well-structured environment provided Mrs Galbraith with a purposeful life. Regularity of habits reduced the problems of incontinence; constipation was prevented by ensuring that she had adequate fluids and a well balanced diet containing fruit, vegetables and fibre.

A programme of planned activities was provided in the ward by the occupational therapist. Mrs Galbraith was encouraged to participate in these activities to meet her need for stimulation; ensuring that she engaged in sufficient activity during the day helped to promote sleep at night. A light supper and a hot drink were given before retiring, and bed time was never too early so that the length of the patient's night was not prolonged beyond normal needs. The provision of a soft light helped to minimise the casting of shadows, and gave Mrs Galbraith a sense of reality on the rare occasions that she did wake up at night.

The nurse cut up Mrs Galbraith's food at mealtimes, because she refused to wear dentures, but she received a normal diet.

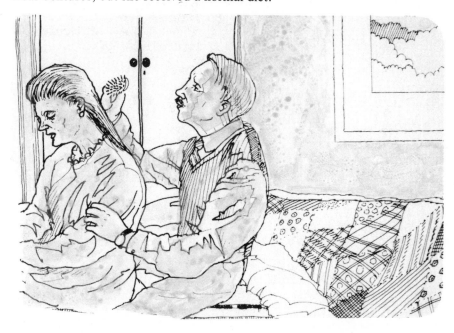

Reality orientation was an essential feature of the geriatric ward: large clocks, calendars and continuous verbal reinforcement helped to impress on Mrs Galbraith where and who she was.

Visiting hours were flexible and the family and friends were welcomed to the ward at any reasonable time. The nurse found she was able to encourage Mrs Galbraith's family to contribute to her care. She knew that the patient's relatives could feel guilty about passing over the caring role to others; she was in a position to alleviate some of these feelings.

One day Mr Galbraith told the nurse, 'My wife had lovely long hair when she was young, nurse, I used to brush it for her', 'Why don't you continue to do that Mr Galbraith' the nurse replied, 'I'm sure your wife would enjoy that'. The nurse was aware that many relatives are happier to be *doing* rather than just sitting down with the patient. The imaginative nurse will think of many ways to encourage family participation, so that they can gain satisfaction from contributing in a useful and meaningful way.

Mrs Galbraith's relatives needed the nurse's support to cope with her changing personality; feelings of sadness may be experienced when the patient is no longer remembered as she used to be. The nurse helps to minimise these changes by preserving the patient's identity.

Rationale

Through the process of caring the nurse promotes the quality of the individual's life.

Evaluation

Mrs Galbraith's care is evaluated at weekly staff meetings. All the nursing objectives have remained operational in promoting the quality and meaningfulness of the patient's life.

Mrs Galbraith's family have accepted that it would not be practicable for her to return home. By allowing them to participate in meeting the patient's needs they feel very much a part of the caring system.

References

1. Eliopoulos, C., *Geriatric Nursing,* Lippincott Nursing Series, Harper & Row, 1979
2. Fish, F., *An Outline of Psychiatry,* Wright, 1964
3. Kastenbaum, R., *Growing Old. Years of Fulfilment.* A Life Cycle Book, Harper & Row, 1979
4. Whitehead, A., In: Hobman, D.(Ed.), *The Social Challenge of Aging,* Croom Helm, 1978

Chapter 11

Nursing the patient who is institutionalised

Introduction

Institutionalisation is a condition which has been recognised as being quite separate from the psychiatric illness which originally initiated the patient's admission to hospital. The condition was first observed among the inmates of various types of institutions; thus the term became established. Institutions are not however the only cause of the condition; some individuals may be institutionalised in their own homes.

The condition was described by Russell Barton[1], who listed the following features:

1. Apathy.
2. Lack of initiative.
3. Loss of interest.
4. Submissiveness.
5. No feelings of resentment.
6. Deterioration of personal habits.
7. Loss of individuality.
8. Resigned acceptance.

The causative factors included loss of contact with the outside world; most psychiatric hospitals were some distance from the nearest town. The travelling and restricted visiting hours at that time added to the difficulties of relatives who wanted to maintain contact with the patient. The nurses themselves fostered dependence rather than independence among patients, and nurses actually prevented patients from carrying out many of the tasks they could do for themselves. Personal events such as birthdays and anniversaries passed unnoticed in the overcrowded wards, and little privacy was to be obtained in the large impersonal dormitories.

Sedatives were often used excessively to control overactive or bizarre behaviour. After years in hospital patients did not welcome the prospect of leaving. They became dependent on the hospital which provided for their basic needs.

Since Russell Barton and others drew attention to the condition of institutionalisation, many changes have taken place in the field of psychiatry and much success has been achieved in the rehabilitation of long-stay patients. One of the most important changes is in the role of the psychiatric nurse: this has in more recent years changed from a custodial to a therapeutic role with greater emphasis being placed on nurse–patient interaction.

Despite the changes, 'new' long-stay patients are still presenting problems today, especially when illness of a chronic nature develops in young people and requires prolonged treatment.

Patient profile

Leah was first admitted to hospital in 1960, with an acute schizophrenic illness; she was then 23. Despite receiving many different kinds of treatment over the years, her behaviour remained disturbed and unpredictable periodically until the mid-1970s. Leah's parents and sister visited her regularly at first, but gradually the visits dwindled away. Both her parents are now dead and her sister, who is married, is unwilling to take Leah into her own home, even for weekend leave.

There has been no evidence of delusions or hallucinations for some time, but Leah maintains that she is not well enough to leave hospital. Her main problem now is that she is institutionalised.

ASSESSMENT INTERVIEW

(Fill in or delete, as appropriate)

Consultant _Dr Peers_

GP _None_

Referred by _____

Date of referral _____ Date of admission _23.4.60_

Short-stay ward _____

Medium-stay ward _____

Long-stay ward _Turner_

Day hospital _____

Community Nursing Service _____

Status _Informal_

Surname ~~Mr/Mrs~~/Miss _Smith_

Forenames _Leah Sarah_

Address _____

Tel. No. _____

Name of next of kin _Mrs cl. Webster (Sister)_

Address _Rose Villas, Hillside, Raylton_

Tel. No. _____

Name by which the patient likes to be addressed _Leah_

Birthday _3.8.37_

DESCRIPTION OF THE PATIENT

Colour of eyes _Green_ Hair colour _Brown/grey_

Height (m) _1.702_ Weight (kg) _77_

Distinguishing features

Ruddy complexion, slight stoop
Wears no dentures

Present occupation/Occupational history

Factory worker prior to admission
Worked in hospital laundry at one time,
now generally helps in the wards, and
attends occupational therapy

Hobbies and interests

Watches television sometimes
Does any jobs or errands for the
nurses

Family or persons of significance in patient's life

Mrs cl. Webster (Sister)
Mother died 1968. Father killed pit accident
_1975_

Persons expected to visit/Support systems

Occasional visit from sister, usually just
before Christmas

Religion

Church of England. Attends hospital
services regularly

Home conditions

Has no home since death of parents

Community services involved/referred

Name of person _None_

Status _____

Tel. No. _____

Whether contacted (and reason for contacting, if relevant)

_____

Psychiatric Condition

Previous psychiatric illness

Schizophrenia. Has not received any
medication for a number of years

Present psychiatric condition

General appearance _An obese woman, who_
takes no interest in her personal
appearance

Behaviour _Co-operative patient, always willing_
to do whatever she is asked. Copes
with routine work and errands on the
ward, shows no other initiative

Speech patterns/content _No evidence of delusion_
or hallucinations now
Doesn't converse with other patients or
staff very much, but will talk when
spoken to

Mood _Placid - never appears to vary_

Orientation _Orientated to immediate_
environment

Patient's understanding of illness _Very little insight._
Believes her parents wanted her out
of the way, and thats why she was
admitted to hospital in the first place

Patient's family's attitudes to patient's illness _Sister visits_
once or perhaps twice a year, move of
a family obligation to their deceased
parents

Present Physical Condition

Result of physical examination

General health good. Overweight

Any physical condition for which the patient is receiving treatment?

None

Activities for daily living

Nutrition

Appetite _Overeats_

Special diet/preferences _Eats anything_

Amount of fluid per day _Approx. 2 litres_

Fluid preferences _Tea or cordial, dislikes coffee_

Elimination

Bowel activity _Regular_

Bladder habit _Regular_

Hygiene

Dentures _Upper plate, refuses to wear it_

Washing   Bathing   Dressing

Needs close supervision in all these areas

Mobility and safety factors

Vision _Normal_

Hearing _Normal_

Sleep patterns _Sleeps well_

Menstrual cycle _N/A_

Areas of concern to the patient (list numerically)

Nothing seems to concern Leah, she says that she is very happy, has no complaints, and wouldn't want to go anywhere else.

Patient's problems identified during interview (list numerically)

1. A lack of interest in events outside the ward environment.
2. Minimal contacts outside the hospital
3. Lacks the initiative to deal with anything other than routine tasks.
4. Never expresses anger or resentment.
5. Lack of social skills apparent at meal times, shows no consideration for other patients; pours water for herself without offering it to other patients; never passes condiments; starts to clear the table before other patients have finished eating.
6. Neglects personal hygiene and appearance, unless instructed to attend to self-care.
7. Content to remain in hospital.

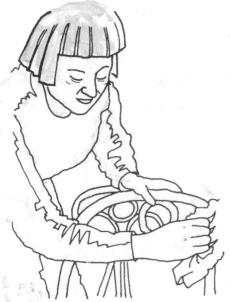

She is co-operative and feels useful because she helps on the ward and runs errands for the nurses. Although she is lax about her personal hygiene and appearance, she will always wash and tidy herself up if told to do so.

Leah is rarely visited by her sister, perhaps once or twice a year. These visits or their infrequency do not seem to worry Leah as she has said that she is very happy in her ward and never wants to leave the hospital.

Plan

1. To encourage the development of social skills.
2. To stimulate Leah's interest in events outside the hospital.
3. To get to know Leah as a person and help her to establish her individuality.
4. To enable her to engage in a self-care programme on her own initiative.
5. To encourage independence.
6. To help her work towards an eventual transition from hospital to community.

Implementation

To encourage the development of social skills, Leah was encouraged to engage in a Token Economy Scheme with a group of other patients. This is a type of behavioural therapy in which tokens or rewards are given for the achievement of desired behaviour. Firstly it was necessary to define the problem areas, i.e. the behaviour which needed to be changed. The staff then agreed the criteria by which to judge the patients' behaviour. The exchange value of tokens and the number to be issued for each type of behaviour were also determined.

Table 11.1 Token economy scheme to achieve short-term goals

Week. . .1. Day. . .4.

Behaviour to be rated	Criteria for acceptance	Token value	Possible target	Satisfies criteria	Unsatis-factory	Daily total
Appearance						
Dress	Garments clean and fastened	1	1	✓		1
Hair	Combed and pinned neatly	1	1	✓		1
Stockings/tights	Pulled up and wrinkle free	1	1		X	—
Shoes	Clean and polished	1	1		X	—
Hygiene						
Mouth care	Cleaning activity is observed	1	2	✓	X	1
Washing/bathing	Hygiene practices observed	1	2	✓		1
Table Manners						
Considers other patients	Offers water	2	6	✓	X X	2
	Passes condiments	2	6	✓	X X	2
	Does not clear table before others have finished eating	2	6	✓✓	X	4

Total 12

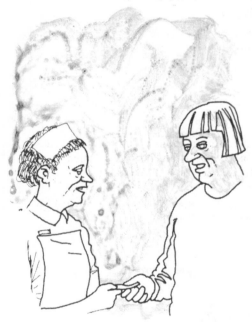

The behaviours designated for change and the criteria for acceptance are listed in Table 11.1. The new type of therapy was introduced to Leah along with some tokens. So that she would appreciate their value in terms of purchasing power it was explained how she could earn more. She was then rewarded, with the agreed tokens, for the achievement of desired behaviour. Each behaviour had to be achieved by Leah's own volition and without any prompting from the nurse. Some activities could earn more tokens than others because it was necessary for them to be performed more frequently. During a six week period Leah's behaviour improved and in the latter weeks she was able to earn up to twenty-two tokens out of a possible daily total of twenty-six. The therapy had succeeded in improving her initiative in as much that she would engage in her own self-care without prompting and her interactions with others had improved during mealtimes.

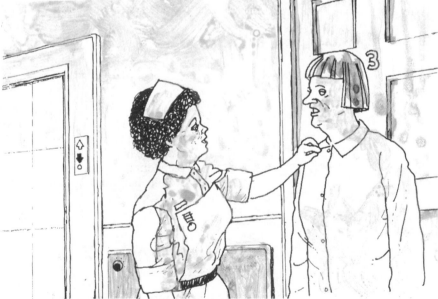

Rationale

As more attention is focused on Leah she will receive the support to enable her to achieve her goals.

Evaluation

The Token Economy Scheme proved successful in providing Leah with an incentive to engage in self-care and to develop some social skills. The nurses must observe Leah to see if she maintains these behaviours now that the Token Scheme has been terminated.

Leah's interest in events outside the hospital is still in need of stimulation; she is being encouraged to read a daily newspaper and discuss current events with the staff. The nurses are getting to know Leah as a person and encouraging her to develop her own individuality by choosing her own clothes and small items for her room.

Leah is gradually being directed towards independence and an eventual life outside the hospital.

More emphasis will now be placed on the patient's attendance at the rehabilitation unit where it is hoped she will acquire the skills for existence in the real world.

Reference

1. Barton, R., *Institutional Neurosis,* Wright, 1959

Chapter 12

Nursing the patient who is dependent on alcohol

Introduction

Individuals who are dependent on drugs or alcohol use these substances as a way of dealing with their problems. Robinson[4] writes that people with addictive personalities do not choose to think their way through problems. They live in their feelings predominantly. They use alcohol and drugs as substitutes for thinking, resolving problems and getting their needs met.

Addiction to drugs and alcohol is a massive world problem; these substances have a deleterious effect on the individual concerned and those closest to him. These substances are taken for a variety of reasons; no single factor can be identified as causative of a person's addiction to drugs or alcohol.

The person who is dependent on alcohol may be seeking solace, comfort or avoidance of facing underlying problems, through this socially acceptable and easily available substance. Irving[2] states that the individual who comes to rely too heavily upon alcohol is generally a dependent person with marked hostility, self-centredness and low frustration tolerance. Usually his dependence is combined with high expectations of himself which he cannot always fulfil.

The dependence is both psychological and physical; the effect of withdrawal of alcohol from the body can result in unpleasant withdrawal symptoms, including tremors, sweating, restlessness, fits, insomnia, aches and pains, vomiting and diarrhoea.

The long-term physical complications resulting from chronic alcoholism include gastric disturbances, liver dysfunction, nutritional deficiencies and neurological changes. These may include memory impairment and dementia.

The pathway to alcoholism is fraught with self-destruction and suffering for both the alcoholic and his family, and meets with negative attitudes from society.

Patient profile

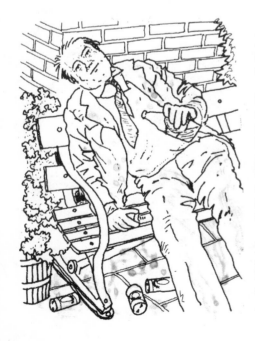

Richard Kimball was 46, married with two teenaged children. He had worked for the same company for a number of years; his own promotion coincided with the company's growth.

Richard had always enjoyed drinking socially, but as his responsibilities increased he began to use alcohol to help him unwind. Then he began to use alcohol to boost his confidence before any important business engagement. At first alcohol gave Richard a sense of well-being and he was able to cope with his business affairs admirably; later he found he needed more and more alcohol to produce the same social performance. Eventually, he was conducting his business on a daily intake of alcohol which would have incapacitated any ordinary drinker. His visits to the pub on the way home from work, his frequent mood changes and irritability severely affected relationships with his wife and children.

Mrs Kimball's salary was essential, and friends were discouraged from visiting the family at home to save any embarrassment. Richard's increasing dependence on alcohol led to frequent absences from work because of sickness. He was asked by his employer to have a medical examination, as a result of which he was persuaded to seek treatment for his condition.

ASSESSMENT INTERVIEW

(Fill in or delete, as appropriate)

Consultant _Dr Issacs_

GP _Dr Glover_

Referred by _GP_

Date of referral _3·9·83_ Date of admission _4·9·83_

Short-stay ward _Hamilton Unit_

Medium-stay ward _____

Long-stay ward _____

Day hospital _____

Community Nursing Service _____

Status _Informal_

Surname Mr/~~Mrs/Miss~~ _Kimball_

Forenames _Richard Carlton_

Address _1A Lower Crescent, Raylton_

Tel. No. _OL 060 2654_

Name of next of kin _Mrs Betty Kimball Wife_

Address _As above_

Tel. No. _____

Name by which the patient likes to be addressed _Richard_

Birthday _16.1.38_

DESCRIPTION OF THE PATIENT

Colour of eyes _Brown_ Hair colour _Dark_

Height (m) _1·829_ Weight (kg) _71·0_

Distinguishing features
Receding hair line, hair brushed close to head

Present occupation/Occupational history
General Manager, Chain Store Group. Promoted from small store over years to present position. Responsibility grown as company grew

Hobbies and interests
Used to like cricket, golf, sailing, reading and theatre. Drinking has taken priority over all these interests

Family or persons of significance in patient's life
Mrs Kimball, children, Malcolm aged 13 and Fiona aged 12

Persons expected to visit/Support systems
Wife and children

Religion
Baptist... Lapsed

Home conditions
Three bedroomed semi-detached house in need of redecoration. Mrs Kimball works full time as a supermarket cashier

Community services involved/referred

Name of person _Alcoholics Anonymous_

Status _____

Tel. No. _060 8876_

Whether contacted (and reason for contacting, if relevant)
Yes

Psychiatric Condition

Previous psychiatric illness
Was treated for anxiety neurosis in 1965 by GP

Present psychiatric condition

General appearance _Has neglected his appearance recently_

Behaviour _Bites nails, smokes 20-30 cigarettes a day_

Speech patterns/content _Hesitant and thoughtful. Told the nurse that he had always lacked confidence in himself_

Mood _Feels tense - on edge all the time. Admits that he has thought about suicide once or twice._

Orientation _Has had blackouts, some clouding of consciousness_

Patient's understanding of illness _Has had difficulty in accepting the diagnosis of alcoholism. Has no real understanding of the harmful effects of alcohol on his body_

Patient's family's attitudes to patient's illness _Wife is very keen for her husband to receive treatment. Says her husband's problem has affected relationships with herself_

Present Physical Condition

Result of physical examination

Myocardial Infarction 7 years ago
Partial gastrectomy 3 years ago
Mild hypertension, iron deficiency anaemia

Any physical condition for which the patient is receiving treatment?

Receives from GP bendrofluazine 5 mg
three times daily, Potassium chloride
500 mg three times daily, Ferrous
sulphate 200 mg three times daily all
taken haphazardly

Activities for daily living

Nutrition

Appetite Only fair, has missed meals
because of drinking

Special diet/preferences Avoids rich spicey
foods since operation

Amount of fluid per day 1½ litres

Fluid preferences Tea 'when on the wagon'

Elimination

Bowel activity Diarrhoea periodically

Bladder habit Increased urinary volume
because of diuretic

Hygiene

Dentures Front teeth capped

Washing Bathing Dressing Needs encouragement
to attend to mouth care, personal hygiene
and general appearance

Mobility and safety factors

Vision Good

Hearing Good

Sleep patterns Restless and poor sleeper

Menstrual cycle N/A

Areas of concern to the patient (list numerically)

Sense of failure - feels he has let his
family down and never really got
to know his children.

Patient's problems identified during interview (list numerically)

1. Feels he has failed himself and his family.
2. Feelings of low esteem.
3. Hostility is present when asked questions about himself.
4. Neglect of self-care.
5. Wants to get better, but is anxious about his ability to cope.
6. Has no understanding of the harmful effects of alcohol on his body.
7. Nutritional deficits caused by alcoholism and poor appetite.
8. Restless and poor sleeper.

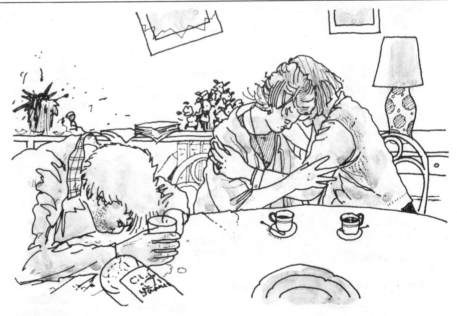

Plan

1. To abstain from alcohol.
2. To accept the patient with understanding and a non-judgemental approach.
3. To ensure that the patient has a clear understanding of the goals of treatment.
4. To ensure that the goals for the patient are realistic and attainable.

5. To reinforce positively the achievement of these goals at every stage of treatment to motivate him towards recovery.
6. To correct nutritional deficits.
7. To increase the patient's sense of self-worth.
8. To encourage him to engage in self-care activities.
9. To educate the patient about the harmful effects of alcohol on his body.
10. To provide a therapeutic environment in which the patient can discuss and gain insight into his problem.
11. To provide cohesive teamwork and support in helping the patient to ventilate his negative feelings.
12. To promote restful sleep.
13. To introduce the patient to Alcoholics Anonymous for continued counselling and support.
14. To communicate with, and engage the support of, the patient's family in achieving the goals of treatment.

Implementation

Primarily if the nurse is to help the patient overcome his addiction to alcohol, she must be prepared to accept him as a worthwhile person, without making moralistic judgements about his behaviour.

Richard was admitted to hospital to obtain medical assistance and for monitoring of his progress during the detoxication period. Fortunately in his case the symptoms caused by the withdrawal of alcohol were not too severe. A minor tranquilliser was prescribed to alleviate some of the discomfort, but this was terminated as soon as it no longer seemed necessary, to avoid the possibility of dependence.

It was essential for Richard and his family to understand the goals of his treatment. The Report of a Special Committee of the Royal College of Psychiatrists on Alcohol and Alcoholism[3] states that clear goals help to relieve the sense of chaos, of 'everything piling in upon him' and make movement towards recovery possible.

In helping to motivate the patient towards recovery the nurse reinforced his achievements. It was essential for the patient to know that he *was* making progress.

Richard had missed many meals during the course of his drinking activities. It was now necessary to ensure that he corrected these nutritional deficits by a well-balanced diet, and that he took prescribed medication regularly to promote his well-being.

He was encouraged to take a pride in his appearance and engage in self-care activities. This helped to increase his self-comfort and self-image. Richard was encouraged to explore his problems in order to gain insight into the reasons for

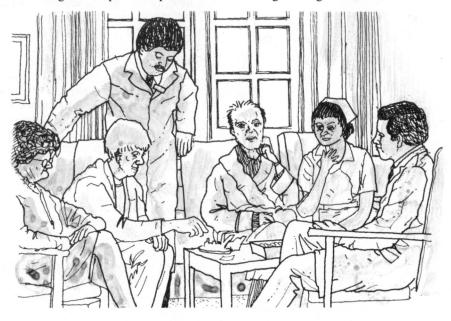

his drinking; this was facilitated through counselling and group therapy. His drinking was never treated as the focus of his problems, and he was guided towards the discovery of the underlying reasons for his addiction.

Self-discovery can be a painful process; at first Richard tried to deny the existence of any problems, at other times he tried to project his feelings of anger onto the nurse.

Topalis and Aguilera[5] write that interpersonal relationships of a therapeutic nature are one of the alcoholic's greatest needs, but the establishment of such relationships is not easy. The major obstacles are the patient's inability to face his own problems and fears, his skilful rationalisation and minimisation of his drinking. . ..

The nurse listened carefully to what Richard had to say and tried to detect areas of concern from his verbal and non-verbal behaviour. It was essential for the nurse to have the support of a cohesive team of colleagues who understood the problems which can arise when caring for the patient who is dependent on alcohol.

One of the nurse's tasks was to educate the patient about the deleterious effects of alcohol on his body. Burgess and Lazare[1] write that the scare approach 'You'll get an enlarged liver', will often lead to a stall situation. The way to correct the stall situation is to use the therapeutic task of setting a goal, such as talking about how alcohol has created difficulties for him personally and his family. The nursing intervention was therefore guided by how the patient perceived his situation. Richard admitted feeling anxious about his health, particularly since he suffered a mild heart attack seven years ago. He learned from the nurse that self-care could do much to reduce the possiblity of disease.

Richard's inability to sleep was reversed through a full programme of activities. Richard was encouraged to develop new interests to fill the time which he had previously occupied by his drinking activities.

Rationale

The nurse assists the patient to gain confidence in his ability to solve his problems without the aid of alcohol.

Evaluation

Richard's progress was evaluated at daily staff meetings. He felt accepted by the staff and demonstrated an understanding of the objectives set for him. His physical condition improved and he experienced less difficulty in sleeping.

Richard learned about the harmful effects of alcohol through the nurse's role as a health educator, gradually gaining some insight into his own behaviour; this self-discovery was facilitated through counselling and group therapy.

Mrs Kimball is pleased with her husband's progress; she has shared his sense of achievement in reaching goals, and is optimistic about the future.

Richard has already been introduced to members of Alcoholics Anonymous who will continue to offer support and counselling when he is discharged.

Before Richard returns to work it will be necessary for the nurse to engage the patient and his family in more long-term goals, if he is to build on the progress already made and maintain his motivation to abstain from alcohol.

These goals must take into consideration the way in which the patient previously coped with his inner needs and his formal social habits.

References

1. Burgess, A.W. and Lazare, A., *Psychiatric Nursing in the Hospital and in the Community,* Prentice Hall, 1976
2. Irving, S., *Basic Psychiatric Nursing,* Saunders, 1978
3. Anon., *Report on Alcohol and Alcoholism of a Special Committee of The Royal College of Psychiatrists,* Tavistock Publications, 1979
4. Robinson, L., *Psychiatric Nursing as a Human Experience,* Saunders, 1977
5. Topalis, M. and Aguilera, D.C., *Psychiatric Nursing,* 7th edn, Mosby, 1978

Fact sheet: Facts about alcohol

Alcohol has a high calorie content but contains no nutrients.

Tests have shown that errors in judgement occur when alcohol is absorbed into the bloodstream.

Alcohol is not an aphrodisiac; increase in sexual desire is due only to a lifting of social inhibitions.

At least half of the injuries suffered in road traffic accidents are caused by alcohol.

Alcohol consumption is not recommended if a person is taking sedatives, tranquillisers, monoamine oxidase inhibitors or antihistamine drugs, or if he suffers from epilepsy, liver disease or gastric ulcer.

Alcohol intoxication is implicated in many instances of suicide, murder and accidental drowning.

Fact sheet: Hangovers

A hangover is a physical condition that follows the consumption of too much alcohol. The main symptoms include a throbbing headache and an upset stomach. The condition is brought about by the following processes:

1. The lining of the stomach being irritated by excessive alcohol.
2. Cell dehydration occurs because the input of alcohol exceeds the liver's ability to process it.
3. The level of alcohol has a shock effect on the central nervous system.

Reference

Diagram Group, *Man's Body,* Paddington Press, 1976

Chapter 13

The use of drugs in psychiatric care

The nurse's role in the giving of medication

The nursing student will already have a knowledge of the rules and regulations regarding the safe storage and administration of medicine. Now she must acquaint herself with some of the drugs commonly used in psychiatric practice. The nurse's role in giving medicine is an important function, and may be beneficial to the patient.

All medicines, whatever their chemical composition, are known to have a placebo effect. The word placebo comes from the latin verb — to please.

Laurence[1] describes a placebo as a vehicle for cure by suggestion; he goes on to say that everyone who administers drugs should be aware that their attitudes to treatment may greatly influence the result. Thus negative attitudes on the nurse's part may prevent a drug from achieving its full effects, whereas positive approaches may potentiate the pharmacological action of a drug.

Often the attitudes of the nurse in hospital may influence the patient's willingness to continue medication when discharged. Wilson Barnett[2] writes that staff can increase adherence to medication among patients by friendly and informative communications with them.

There is no doubt that drugs have brought about revolutionary changes and new dimensions to the care of the mentally ill, enabling many patients to live useful and fulfilling lives in the community.

While such preparations are important in relieving the patient's symptoms and aiding his recovery the nurse should never consider drugs to be a *substitute* for effective nursing care.

A list of some of the more common drugs used in the management of psychiatric illness is given below, but this is not intended to be a comprehensive list and the student should consult a suitable pharmacology textbook.

(a) An important note

- No medicines should be taken except those prescribed by a doctor.
- Should the patient require either a local or general anaesthetic, the anaesthetising officer must be informed of the patient's medication.

References

1. Laurence, M.D., *Clinical Pharmacology*, Churchill Livingstone, 1973
2. Wilson Barnett, J., *Stress in Hospital — Patient's Psychological Reactions to Illness and Health Care*, Churchill Livingstone, 1979

Psychotropic drugs

Psychotropic drugs are a common feature of the patient's treatment, therefore the nurse must have a sound knowledge regarding patient's medications.

The nurse must know:

1. The dosage range of the medication.
2. The specific action of the medication and its therapeutic effectiveness.
3. The side effects.
4. Ways in which side effects are alleviated.
5. Prohibited foods or drugs which may react adversely with the prescribed medication.
6. Precautions which must be taken to maintain the patient's safety and well-being in carrying out his daily activities, e.g. drowsiness which could inhibit driving ability.

through carelessness or ignorance, increase any risk to his well-being.

Further reading

Boettcher, E. and Alderson, S.F., Psychotropic drugs and the nursing process, *Journal of Psychosocial Nursing and Mental Health Services,* **20**, No. 11, Nov., 1982
Laurence, D.R., *Clinical Pharmacology,* 4th edn, Churchill Livingstone, 1973

Suggested reading

BOOKS WHICH SPECIFICALLY DEAL WITH DRUGS USED IN PSYCHIATRY
Crammer, J., Barraclough, B. and Heine, B., *The Use of Drugs in Psychiatry,* Gaskell Books, 1978
Silverstone, T. and Turner, P., *Drug Treatment in Psychiatry,* Routledge and Kegan Paul, 1978

A MORE GENERAL TEXTBOOK
Turner, P. and Richens, A., *Clinical Pharmacology,* 3rd edn, Churchill Livingstone, 1978

Tables 13.1 – 13.7 list the more common drugs used in psychiatry.

Table 13.1   Major tranquillisers

Approved name	Trade name	Recommended dose	Uses	Side effects
Chlorpromazine	Largactil	25–500 mg three times daily	Has a general calming effect. Reduces psychomotor activity. Used in schizophrenia and affective disorders. Relieves anxiety and agitation. Suppresses delusions and hallucinations	Postural hypotension; photosensitivity, hypothermia; blood dyscrasias; blurring of vision. Dryness of mouth. Constipation. Skin rashes. Parkinson-like syndrome. Drowsiness. Potentiate the action of other drugs.
Perphenazine	Fentazin	2–15 mg three times daily	As above	As above
Promazine	Sparine	25–100 mg three times daily	Particularly useful in senile agitation and alcoholism	As above
Prochlorperazine	Stemetil	Up to 100 mg daily	Used in mind emotional disturbances	As above but usually less severe
Thiopropazate	Dartalan	15–30 mg daily	Psychosis and psychoneurosis. May relieve symptoms of dyskinesia	As chlorpromazine
Thiothixene	Navane	75–150 mg daily	For schizophrenia, not as effective as chlorpromazine	Prone to cause extrapyramidal symptoms
Trifluoperazine	Stelazine	2–30 mg daily	Schizophrenia. Psychoses due to brain damage. Chronic alcoholism	As chlorpromazine. Extrapyramidal symptoms likely
Thioridazine	Melleril	10–200 mg three times daily	Effective in relieving agitation and restlessness	As chlorpromazine. Retinal pigmentation in prolonged doses
Haloperidol	Serenace	1–12 mg daily	Effective in controlling excitement and overactivity in schizophrenia and mania	As chlorpromazine. Prone to cause extrapyramidal symptoms and depression
Trifluoperidol	Triperdol	1–3 mg daily	Effective in schizophrenia and manic depressive psychoses	As above, depression less likely

Table 13.2 *Anti-Parkinsonian drugs*

Approved name	Trade name	Recommended dose	Uses	Side effects
Benzhexol	Artane	5–15 mg daily	*Common to this group* Anti-Parkinsonian drugs are given to relieve extrapyramidal symptoms	*Common to this group* Drowsiness. Nausea. Dry mouth. Constipation. Urinary difficulties
Benzetropine	Cogentin	0.5–6 mg daily		
Procyclidine	Kemadrin	10–30 mg daily		
Orphenadrine	Disipal	100–300 mg daily		

Table 13.3 *Minor tranquillisers*

Approved name	Trade name	Recommended dose	Uses	Side effects
Chlordiazepoxide	Librium	10–100 mg daily	Relieves anxiety and tension. Muscle relaxant	Drowsiness. Dizziness. Constipation. Ataxia. Appetite stimulant. Anticonvulsant in higher doses
Diazepam	Valium	4–80 mg daily	As above	As above

Table 13.4 *Long-acting tranquillisers*

Approved name	Trade name	Recommended dose	Uses	Side effects
Flupenthixol decanoate	Depixol	20–100 mg every 2–4 weeks	Used for anxiety, depression, schizophrenia, mania and atypical illnesses	Extrapyramidal effects are less common. Overactivity can occur
Fluphenazine enanthate	Moditen enanthate	12.5–25 mg every 1–4 weeks	Highly suitable for long-term out-patient treatment of chronic schizophrenia and for patients who are suspicious of tablets	Side effects may require anti-Parkinsonian drugs
Fluphenazine decanoate	Modecate	12.5–25 mg every 2–4 weeks	As above	Drowsiness and flattening of affect may occur

Table 13.5 *Tricyclic antidepressants*

Approved name	Trade name	Recommended dose	Uses	Side effects
Imipramine	Tofranil	100–200 mg daily	*Common to this group* Used for endogenous depression. Less effective for reactive depression	*Common to this group* Dry mouth. Blurred vision. Sweating. Restlessness. Tachycardia. Hypotension. Urinary retention. Tremor. Gastro intestinal upsets. Blood dyscrasias. Ataxia. Vertigo
Amitriptyline	Tryptizol	10–25 mg three times daily or 150 mg daily		
Nortriptyline	Aventyl	25 mg daily		
Protriptyline	Concordin	10 mg two to four times daily or 20 mg three times daily		
Trimipramine	Surmontil	75–300 mg daily 75–150 mg maintenance		
Dothiepin	Prothiaden	25–50 mg three times daily		
Clomipramine	Anafranil	50–150 mg daily 50–100 mg maintenance dose		

Table 13.6 Monoamine oxidase inhibitors

Approved name	Trade name	Recommended dose	Uses	Side effects
			Common to this group	*Common to this group*
Phenelzine	Nardil	15–30 mg three times daily	Monoamine oxidase inhibitors increase brain amine levels which are reduced in depression	Postural hypotension. Giddiness. Headaches. Blurred vision. Skin rashes. Liver damage. Impotence. Severe hypertensive crisis if amine-rich foods are taken*
Isocarboxazid	Marplan	30 mg a day in divided doses		
Iproniazid	Marsilid	100–150 mg daily 25–50 mg maintenance		
Nialamide	Niamid	75–150 mg daily in divided doses		
Tranycypromine	Parnate	10 mg two or three times daily		

*Foods containing tyramine are prohibited from the patient's diet. Patients receiving monoamine oxidase inhibitors are given a card which lists the foods which should be omitted from the diet. These foods may include: alcohol, cheese, broad beans, bananas, meat and yeast extracts, pickled herrings, chicken liver.

Table 13.7 Other drugs

Approved name	Trade name	Recommended dose	Uses	Side effects
Lithium carbonate	Priadel	1200–1600 mg daily	Used in manic depressive psychosis	Diarrhoea. Vomiting. Tremor. Fatigue. Gastrointestinal disturbances*

* Regular monitoring of blood serum essential.

Further reading

Aslam, M. and Stockley, I.H., Drugs in psychiatry, *Nursing Times,* Sept. 6, 1979

Crammer, J., Barraclough, B. and Heine, B., *The Use of Drugs in Psychiatry,* Gaskell Books, 1978

Silverstone, T. and Turner, P., *Drug Treatment in Psychiatry,* Routledge and Kegan Paul, 1974

Chapter 14   Exercises

From the following patient profiles and assessment interviews:

1. Identify the patient's problems.
2. Set goals for the patient which will help him/her overcome these problems.
3. Describe the nursing intervention which will be necessary to help the patient reach these goals.
4. How will you evaluate the achievement of these goals?

After attempting these exercises you may check the outcome with the answer guides which follow them.

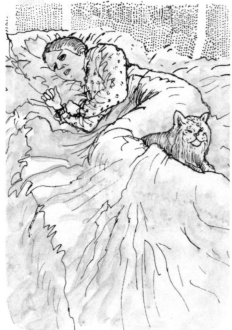

Patient profile

Sarah Brown, aged 32, has lived with her mother since divorcing her husband three years ago.

She enjoyed her work as a window dresser in a large London store, but the recession meant that many firms had to make cutbacks, and Sarah was made redundant. Sarah's search for similar work has so far proved unsuccessful, making her feel thoroughly disheartened and depressed. Her self-confidence has been severely shaken.

Although Sarah normally gets on well with her mother, she now finds her company irritating. Mrs Lloyd, who was sympathetic when her daughter was made redundant, feels now that she should pull herself together.

After visiting her GP, and complaining of feeling low and run down, Sarah was referred to the Community Psychiatric Nurse, who was asked to visit Sarah and provide support.

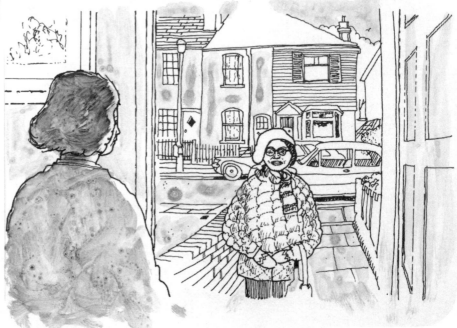

ASSESSMENT INTERVIEW

(Fill in or delete, as appropriate)

Consultant _____
GP _____ Dr Pitt _____
Referred by _____ GP _____
Date of referral _13.6.83_ Date of admission _____
Short-stay ward _____
Medium-stay ward _____
Long-stay ward _____
Day hospital _____
Community Nursing Service _____
Status _____

Surname ~~Mr/Mrs/Miss~~ _Brown_
Forenames _Sarah Louise_
Address _A Meadowfield Drive_
Raylton

Tel. No. _____ 01 060 1427 _____
Name of next of kin _Mrs D Lloyd_
Address _Same address_

Tel. No. _____
Name by which the patient likes to be addressed _Sarah_
Birthday _____ 25.11.50 _____

DESCRIPTION OF THE PATIENT
Colour of eyes _Grey and Green_ Hair colour _Auburn_
Height (m) _1.524_ Weight (kg) _38.1_

Distinguishing features
One eye grey, the other green

Present occupation/Occupational history
After basic education, attended
Art College. Worked as a window
dresser for a large London Store.
Made redundant two months ago
Hobbies and interests
Painting and drawing, cooking,
needlework and swimming

Family or persons of significance in patient's life
Mother.
Has several close friends

Persons expected to visit/Support systems

Religion
None

Home conditions
Lives with mother (stepfather dead)
in a pleasant two-bedroomed house

Community services involved/referred
Name of person _Mrs Christine Smith_
Status _Community Psychiatric Nurse_
Tel. No. _____ 01 060 1480 _____
Whether contacted (and reason for contacting, if relevant)
Referred to provide support

Psychiatric Condition

Previous psychiatric illness
Saw child psychiatrist while at school.
Sarah was twelve when her father died,
she attempted to drown herself
following his death
Present psychiatric condition
General appearance _Appears depressed_
and anxious

Behaviour _Has avoided contact with others_
by remaining in bed.
Seems tense, smokes incessantly

Speech patterns/content _Voice is flat, but is_
willing to talk about the way she feels.
Says that she will never try and do
something silly

Mood _Feels dejected in the mornings_
particularly, but a little brighter as the
day goes on. Cries quite a lot when alone
Orientation _Normal_

Patient's understanding of illness _Accepts that she_
is suffering from a depressive illness

Patient's family's attitudes to patient's illness _Mother is_
concerned and sympathic but feels
Sarah should pull herself together

Present Physical Condition

Result of physical examination

General health good

Any physical condition for which the patient is receiving treatment?

None

Activities for daily living

Nutrition

Appetite _Tends to overeat when depressed_

Special diet/preferences _Likes most things_

Amount of fluid per day _1½ – 2 litres_

Fluid preferences _Tea or coffee_

Elimination

Bowel activity _Regular_

Bladder habit _Normal_

Hygiene

Dentures _Upper plate_

Washing Bathing Dressing

Engages in self-care activities

Mobility and safety factors

Vision _Wears glasses for reading_

Hearing _Good_

Sleep patterns _Usually gets up and makes a cup of tea during the night – has difficulty getting back to sleep_

Menstrual cycle _Regular until recently_

Areas of concern to the patient (list numerically)

Very concerned about getting another job as a window dresser.

Patient's problems identified during interview (list numerically)

Answer guide

Sarah Brown

Sarah's feelings of depression most probably relate to her loss of employment and subsequently the loss of a creative activity that she enjoyed doing.

Her present feeling of loss may have aroused similar feelings caused through the break up of her marriage; similarly on her father's death. Feelings of low esteem most likely account for Sarah's avoidance of others by remaining in bed.

The individual who is depressed frequently harbours a desire to hide herself away, because she perceives herself as less worthwhile.

The patient tried to drown herself when she was 12 years old, yet she has reassured the nurse that she would never do anything silly again. The nurse can never accept such a statement of reassurance. Indeed, the patient may be expressing that suicidal thoughts *are* going through her mind. The nurse can best help the patient by her willingness to listen and share the patient's problems. The nurse must always bear in mind that a depressed patient may be potentially suicidal. Sarah's mother, though sympathetic, feels that her daughter should pull herself together. Some people are unable to appreciate that the depressed person cannot just snap out of their mood. A more positive and constructive approach would be more helpful to Sarah. The nurse could try and change Mrs Lloyd's attitude by increasing her knowledge of depressive illness.

Sarah's tendency to comfort herself by overeating is not usually harmful, and she should overcome this as her mood lifts and she gains insight into her problems.

It is important for the patient who is depressed to have something to do. Most Community Psychiatric Nurses have access to clubs and other facilities which can provide support and activities to aid the patient's recovery.

In the present economic climate, Sarah may be unable to obtain window dressing or similar work. The nurse may have to guide Sarah towards considering other alternatives.

Patient profile

Peter Irons, aged 20, although never a good mixer had shown promise at school, and left with good grades in 'O' and 'A' levels. Following a successful interview in which he had to compete with several other candidates he obtained a job as a trainee manager with a large London chain store. The post necessitated Peter finding digs in London; he managed to get home most weekends to see his family. One weekend when Peter was expected he failed to arrive, and Mrs Irons telephoned his digs to find out what had happened. She was told that he had moved out several days previously without giving any forwarding address.

The following Monday Mrs Irons rang Peter's employers and found that he had not been to work for two weeks; they were concerned as to Peter's whereabouts. Mrs Irons telephoned later in the week to see if they had heard anything; the answer was no. She asked if they were satisfied with Peter, and if they could throw any light on his disappearance. Mrs Voss, the personnel officer, replied that recently Peter had been warned over his general attitude. He appeared to lack any interest in his job, was frequently missing from his department and found to be walking around other parts of the store as if in a dream. There was no news of Peter for three months; efforts to find him proved fruitless.

On returning from shopping one morning Mrs Irons saw a dishevelled figure sitting on the doorstep; it was Peter, although barely recognisable. His behaviour was strange; he didn't even greet his mother and she couldn't find out anything of his whereabouts over the last few months.

Peter's parents found his strange withdrawn behaviour completely out of character and difficult to cope with. The GP was asked to visit and duly arranged for Peter to be admitted to a psychiatric hospital, where a schizophrenic illness was diagnosed.

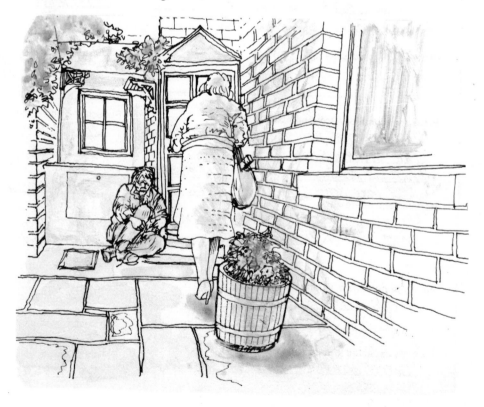

ASSESSMENT INTERVIEW

(Fill in or delete, as appropriate)

Consultant _Dr Foster_

GP _Dr Singh_

Referred by _GP_

Date of referral _____ Date of admission _____

Short-stay ward _Landseer Ward_

Medium-stay ward _____

Long-stay ward _____

Day hospital _____

Community Nursing Service _____

Status _Informal_

Surname Mr/~~Mrs/Miss~~ _Irons_

Forenames _Peter Andrew_

Address _51 Tudor Rise, Raylton_

_____

Tel. No. _01 060 1519_

Name of next of kin _Mr and Mrs J Irons (Parents)_

Address _As above_

_____

Tel. No. _____

Name by which the patient likes to be addressed _Peter_

Birthday _1.4.62_

DESCRIPTION OF THE PATIENT

Colour of eyes _Hazel_   Hair colour _Black_

Height (m) _1.626_   Weight (kg) _60.3_

Distinguishing features

Acne

_____

Present occupation/Occupational history

Has worked as a trainee manager, chain store London since leaving school. Lost his position when he went absent without trace some three months ago

Hobbies and interests

Has always been keen on reading, tennis and visiting museums.

_____

Family or persons of significance in patient's life

Parents and sister, mother's two sisters

_____

Persons expected to visit/Support systems

Parents and sister, one aunt (other bedridden)

Religion

Church of England

Home conditions

Returned to parent's detached house four days ago. Whereabouts not known since leaving digs in London three months ago

Community services involved/referred

Name of person _Mrs Christine Smith_

Status _Community Psychiatric Nurse_

Tel. No. _01 060 1480_

Whether contacted (and reason for contacting, if relevant)

Referred for follow up

Psychiatric Condition

Previous psychiatric illness

None. No history of mental illness in the family. Mrs Irons has never met her husband's family and says he is mysterious about his background

Present psychiatric condition

General appearance _Neglected and unshaven. Maintains a blank facial expression but smiles to himself occasionally_

Behaviour _Sits or stands around motionless. Posture and gait stiff. Withdraws from contact with others_

Speech patterns/content _Words are few 'I'm on a mission... They have contacted me'_

Mood _Mood seems flat and unresponsive_

Orientation _Seems confused and perplexed_

Patient's understanding of illness _Difficult to ascertain_

Patient's family's attitudes to patient's illness _Both parents seem very concerned_

Present Physical Condition

Result of physical examination

General health good. Mouth ulcers due to poor oral hygiene

Any physical condition for which the patient is receiving treatment?

No

Activities for daily living

Nutrition

Appetite *Eats well but mealtime behaviour is poor*

Special diet/preferences *Doesn't eat liver*

Amount of fluid per day *1 litre*

Fluid preferences *Milk*

Elimination

Bowel activity *Regular*

Bladder habit *Normal*

Hygiene

Dentures *None*

Washing Bathing Dressing
Requires supervision with these activities

Mobility and safety factors

Vision *Good*

Hearing *Good*

Sleep patterns *Sleeps soundly*

Menstrual cycle *N/A*

Areas of concern to the patient (list numerically)

Difficult to ascertain on admission

Patient's problems identified during interview (list numerically)

Answer guide

Peter Irons

The nurse's first task will be to try and establish a relationship with the patient. This may take considerable time and effort because Peter has withdrawn from contact with others. Therefore the nurse must be prepared to communicate with Peter both verbally and non-verbally, without threatening him and making him retreat into himself even more.

From observing Peter's behaviour, it is most likely that he is deluded and hallucinated. The nurse must not reinforce these symptoms, she must however record accurately any statements the patient makes which signify his delusions and observe his behaviour in response to hallucinatory experiences.

When encouraging Peter to engage in self-care activities the nurse must try to ensure that he pays particular attention to skin cleansing and regularly washes his face with soap and water. Peter will also need a well-balanced diet with adequate vitamins and protein. His mealtime behaviour will most likely improve as he becomes more aware of the presence of others.

Mr and Mrs Irons will need the nurse's support and understanding, and the Community Psychiatric Nurse should establish rapport with Peter and his family at the earliest opportunity.

Schizophrenia can bring with it special problems of management for the patient's relatives; the nurse can do much to alleviate the relatives' fears by helping them to cope with the patient's behaviour.

Index